PRAISE ~~FOR LIVING~~ LARGE

"Having been a 'skinny guy' growing up, I wish I'd had Vince's *Living Large* to guide me. It would have saved me years of frustrating trial and error. Vince knows his stuff and is not only a great teacher when it comes to building muscle, he's also an ongoing student, always ~~...~~ Big' column in *Iron Man* was always the one I looked for ~~...~~ -solid muscle-building info— and he continues that with ~~...~~

~~...~~ IEF, *IRON MAN* MAGAZINE

"Vince Del Monte is a worth ~~...~~ He's been there and earned every pound. This book will ~~...~~

—SEAN HYSON ~~...~~ *LE & FITNESS* MAGAZINES

"Vince has put together an e ~~...~~ atural way. His programming is easy to follow but brutally ~~...~~ ement these methods I have no doubt that you will make ~~...~~

~~...~~ CTOR FOR *MEN'S HEALTH*

"Anyone who's ever wanted ~~...~~ benefit from Vince's simple, no-nonsense approach to b ~~...~~

—MARK SISSO ~~...~~ MARKSDAILYAPPLE.COM

"As a how-to guide, this b ~~...~~ orward strategies anyone can use to overcome the ~~...~~ d dominating live."

~~...~~ STRENGTH CAMP GYM

"If I could have a personal ~~...~~ my side. Since we live in different countries, this is ~~...~~ lthy size that lasts!"

—LEWIS HOWES, *NEW Y* ~~...~~ GREATNESS" PODCAST

"Getting bigger isn't alway ~~...~~

~~...~~ F EVIDENCEMAG.COM

"Vince is known worldwide ~~...~~ undreds of thousands of men not only build the bo ~~...~~ l them to live large. Vince is more than just a ripped ~~...~~ y to build muscle (even if you think you're doomed ~~...~~ in all areas of your life. If you're a man, this is a mus ~~...~~

—YURI ELKAIM, *NEW YORK TIMES* BESTSELLING AUTHOR
OF *THE ALL-DAY ENERGY DIET* AND *THE ALL-DAY FAT-BURNING DIET*

"Vince writes in an engaging, conversational style that doesn't undersell the difficulty of adding 30 pounds of muscle, but provides all the tools to make it happen. *Living Large* is a solid introduction to building a solid physique."

—LOU SCHULER, COAUTHOR OF THE NEW RULES OF LIFTING SERIES

"Frankly, it doesn't matter how much muscle you build with Vince's advice, whether it's 30 pounds in 30 weeks or just the extra 10 you need for the perfect body. . . . That pales in comparison to what you will REALLY get from the book, and that's the confidence and attitude you need to Live Large, get the girl of your dreams, and leave the legacy for your life. That is his true gift to you. Vince has long been a mentor and role model to me, and I highly recommend you make him the top one in your life today, too."

—CRAIG BALLANTYNE, AUTHOR OF *THE PERFECT DAY FORMULA*

"I've known Vince for over a decade . . . and he is definitely not a fitness meathead. He's a husband, father of two, and extremely successful guy who uses his physical accomplishments of living large inside the gym to inspire others to live large outside of the gym. Vince shows that muscle can be the 'silver bullet' to getting whatever else you want in life . . . whether it be a career, relationship, or lifestyle enhancement . . . and this is the ultimate guide to show you exactly how to do just that."

—BEN GREENFIELD, AUTHOR OF THE *NEW YORK TIMES* BESTSELLER
BEYOND TRAINING: MASTERING ENDURANCE, HEALTH, & LIFE

"I have known Vince for a period of over 5 years. In that time I have been continually amazed at the thoroughness of Vince's approach to building muscle. Rather than use old-school bro science, Vince is willing to delve into actual science first and then create a program from this. Using the perfect mixture of personal experience and research, Vince has created a groundbreaking new book that is virtually fail-proof. The reason I say that is because it is designed to be flexible to your needs and your genetic makeup. I fully endorse this book!"

—DR. JACOB WILSON, CEO OF THE APPLIED SCIENCE AND PERFORMANCE INSTITUTE

"For nearly 30 years, I've been in the 'muscle game.' The last 15 I've had the joy of watching Vince grow from a skinny kid, eager to learn, to the hulking, strong, wise master teacher of the muscle game he is. In your own quest for the perfect physique you will be sent down many dead-end roads by wanna-be gurus. Please, spare yourself the wasted years and money and grab this intelligent guide to muscle and a full strength life. When Vince speaks, listen. For he speaks the truth earned in the trenches, with blood, sweat and iron."

—SHAWN PHILLIPS, "THE PHILOSOPHER OF FIT" AND AUTHOR OF *STRENGTH FOR LIFE* AND *ABSOLUTION*

"When it comes to health and fitness, Vince Del Monte is a forward thinker. Vince knows what it takes to keep the body healthy and allow you to train at a high level. Through his thought process, Vince prepares clients to optimize their fitness goals. Utilizing the components of exercise and recovery discussed in *Living Large* will enable you the opportunity to maximize your health gains."

—GREG ROSKOPF, DEVELOPER AND FOUNDER OF MUSCLE ACTIVATION TECHNIQUES

"*Living Large* is one of the few books I've seen on gaining solid development that not only provides a detailed workout program, exercises, and meal plans, but also really digs deep into the actual mindset that will produce an excellent physique, which is in line with most of my own writings as well. (I especially liked the section 'Focus on Habits, Not Outcomes.') In its discussion of the workout program, the book focuses on going beyond moving the weight from point A to point B, but also on getting the most out of every rep of every exercise. In short, this is a book from someone who has put in his time in the weight room, and who respects both the art and the science of bodybuilding."

—SCOTT ABEL, AUTHOR OF *THE HARDGAINER SOLUTION*

"Vince Del Monte is the ultimate coach for that special breed of people who are willing to take a no-nonsense approach to their training and life. This book simply delivers! For anyone who has been wasting their time in the gym and wants everything to build muscle in one spot, this is it. You're going to get the 30-week DTS muscle-building program and much more and how to execute every single rep for maximum results! The best part? The *Living Large* principles are timeless."

—MATT STIRLING, WBFF PRO AND THREE-TIME WORLD BODYBUILDING CHAMPION

"We need more specialists and fewer 'jacks of all trades.' Most fitness plans lack the focus needed for body transformation. *Living Large* is a realistic plan on a realistic schedule for real results that last. No false hype or 4-week promises. Vince uses the best equation: hard work + great plans that work."

—ADAM BORNSTEIN, *NEW YORK TIMES* BESTSELLING AUTHOR AND FOUNDER OF BORN FITNESS

"*Living Large* is a concise, step-by-step process that will help the hardgainer build muscle. The training and eating programs are easy to follow and there are a ton of useful tips and tricks to ensure your success."

—DR. KEN KINAKIN DC, CSCS, FOUNDER OF THE SOCIETY OF WEIGHT-TRAINING INJURY SPECIALISTS

"Vince Del Monte's *Living Large* is one of the absolute best books I have ever read on gaining muscle. Vince maps the entire process out in a series of simple-to-follow methods and techniques that will help any person achieve serious gains in the fastest time possible. I only wish I had this valuable resource when I was starting out! If you want a no-BS approach to transforming your body, this is it."

—BRUCE KRAHN, AUTHOR OF *TROUBLE SPOT FAT LOSS* AND *THE FAT-FIGHTER DIET*

"If you're scrawny, you need to read this book, the info is out-of-this-world good. The real gem, however, is in Vince's approach to life and the mind-set required to 'live large.' When you get a chance to get into the mind of someone like Vince, take it. It's an awesome read, a rite of passage for any skinny on his way to big things."

—CHAD HOWSE, AUTHOR OF *THE MAN DIET*

"A genuine advantage for any guy serious about gaining his first 30 pounds of muscle. *Living Large* would have saved me years of frustration as a scrawny hardgainer."

—SCOTT TOUSIGNANT, CREATOR OF METABOLIC MASTERPIECE

"If you're a skinny guy looking to build muscle, this book is going to be your new best friend . . . your roadmap to serious muscle and strength and the body you want. Vince has done a phenomenal job not only with the physical aspect of training for muscle growth, but the all-important mental aspect as well (which honestly, can be even harder to master than the physical). Get this book, follow the step-by-step program, and succeed."

—NICK NILSSON, CREATOR OF MAD SCIENTIST MUSCLE

"Vince truly brings exceptional passion, knowledge, and motivation to the table in this book. Vince has spent years learning from and surrounding himself with the top experts in the field in regards to exercise, nutrition, and supplementation. He has been able to marry both the science and practical application into one piece. Vince doesn't just talk the talk but he walks the walk and pushes himself each and every day to be better and live larger. This book is a gem to be treasured and a must to share with friends and family."

—RYAN LOWERY, PRESIDENT OF THE APPLIED SCIENCE AND PERFORMANCE INSTITUTE

"If there's a unifying characteristic of Vince's decade's worth of articles on Bodybuilding.com, it is that he consistently overdelivers. *Living Large* continues the trend. The programming is rock solid, Vince's perspective is spot-on, and you get to eat the egg yolks. What more do you want? This is how you'll grow."

—NICK COLLIAS, DEPUTY EDITOR OF BODYBUILDING.COM

"I LOVE it when I come across powerfully effective fitness advice that comes from an amazing person oozing tremendous energy—who is also successful in all areas of life. That's when you KNOW you'll be able to actually follow through with everything you learn and use it forever. Vince Del Monte's *Living Large* is a welcomed and much-needed source of information in this world filled with impractical advice from fitness extremists who only think about their bodies all day long."

—SKIP LA COUR, SIX-TIME NATIONAL DRUG-FREE BODYBUILDING CHAMPION AND SUCCESS COACH

"Vince Del Monte has incredibly rare talent: he makes a complex process simple to understand without trying to trick the reader into thinking it'll be simple to achieve. All the while, he provides the tools necessary to shorten the learning curve and build an impressive body in record time. *Living Large* is a masterwork of knowledge, insight, and balance; one that will easily earn a place in the library of any training enthusiast, from gym newbies to seasoned fitness pro."

—JOHN ROMANIELLO, *NEW YORK TIMES* BESTSELLING AUTHOR OF *ENGINEERING THE ALPHA*

"Vince Del Monte has created a very solid resource with the release of his book *Living Large*. He blends a good amount of evidence-based science, with real world, in-the-gym training advice. If you read this book, you are sure to walk away with some great takeaways."

—GREGORY O'GALLAGHER, FOUNDER OF KINOBODY.COM

"Vince Del Monte is a man who practices what he preaches! I have known Vince for many years and what I love about him is that he lives what he speaks and writes about; he was the skinny kid who was treated poorly and who knows, first hand, just how it can negatively affect a man's life. . . . As a fellow published author of over 30 books and 2 million copies sold, I applaud Vince and his obvious passion for wanting to truly help men become their very best. I don't typically ever endorse other writers, simply because I never know if they are the 'real deal' and don't want my name attached to people who are simply in it for a 'quick fix.' Vince has been at this for many years, has achieved tremendous success, and will be here, helping people, for years to come. Bravo on writing a wonderful book, Vince. Your book will surely help many men learn how to finally begin living LARGE!"

—JAMES VILLEPIGUE, BESTSELLING AUTHOR OF THE BODY SCULPTING BIBLE FRANCHISE

"If you want proven techniques the pros use to get results, read closely. In *Living Large*, you'll learn how to harness the power of muscle damage, mechanical tension, and metabolic stress in a progressive, step-by-step program. Put these strategies to work and you'll be a superhero in no time."

—ABEL JAMES, NEW YORK TIMES BESTSELLING AUTHOR OF *THE WILD DIET*

"Building muscle can be one of the most challenging goals regardless of your experience level, age, or genes. What I love about Vince is his confidence to hit the reset button and rethink muscle growth. In the years that I have known Vince he has never stopped learning and never stopped educating himself— he is truly a student of muscle building. If you're looking for a simple, smart, and strategic approach to building muscle, then don't miss out."

—BRAD PILON, AUTHOR OF *EAT STOP EAT*

"Amazing but true . . . people really did call him 'Skinny Vinny.' But with discipline and determination, Vince transformed himself and is living large in every way. Even more, he's helped thousands of other guys transform themselves, too. Honestly, if you put the lessons in this book to work for you, you'll gain muscle, confidence, and live a richer life."

—DR. JOHN BERARDI, COFOUNDER OF PRECISION NUTRITION

"I sure do wish I had this book when I started clanging the weights as a twelve-year-old! I would have made a lot more progress in my training, prevented a lot of injuries, and saved a lot of wasted time. Vince has produced a one-of-a-kind masterpiece with *Living Large* and when he asked me to review it, I simply couldn't put it down. Vince cuts through ALL of the industry BS and gives you the no-nonsense TRUTH about training hard to build muscle. No wonder they call him the 'Skinny Guy Savior!' I have had the pleasure of knowing Vince for several years now and he never ceases to amaze me with his ability to distill very complex concepts into simple and easy-to-understand instructions. This book is your step-by-step blueprint of how to gain the most muscle mass possible in the shortest amount of time. Vince lays out the science behind muscle building, but in a manner that those of us who don't live in lab coats all day can understand, and learning the power of optimizing D-T-S (you'll know what that means when you crack open the book) is the key to unlocking your muscular potential. This is, in my opinion, the best muscle-building book of all time!"

—RYAN FAEHNLE, INTERNATIONAL STRENGTH AND PERFORMANCE COACH

LIVING LARGE

LIVING LARGE

THE SKINNY GUY'S GUIDE TO NO-NONSENSE MUSCLE BUILDING

VINCE DEL MONTE

BenBella Books, Inc.
Dallas, TX

BenBella Books, Inc.
PO Box 572028
Dallas, TX 75357-2028
www.benbellabooks.com
Send feedback to feedback@benbellabooks.com

Printed in Malaysia
10 9 8 7 6 5 4 3 2 1

Library of Congress Cataloging-in-Publication Data is available upon request.
978-1-941631-82-9

Editing by Heather Butterfield and Eryn Carlson
Copyediting by Karen Levy
Proofreading by Sarah Vostok and Jenny Bridges
Text design and composition by Kit Sweeney
Front cover design by Ty Nowicki
Full cover design by Sarah Dombrowsky
Cover and interior photography by Arsenik Studios Inc.
Printed by Tien Wah Press

Distributed by Perseus Distribution
www.perseusdistribution.com

To place orders through Perseus Distribution:
Tel: (800) 343-4499
Fax: (800) 351-5073
E-mail: orderentry@perseusbooks.com

Special discounts for bulk sales (minimum of 25 copies) are available.
Please contact Aida Herrera at aida@benbellabooks.com.

To my B.M.W., a.k.a. my beautiful, marvelous wife
for supporting me in living larger inside *and* outside of the gym!

YOUR FREE ONLINE VIDEO COURSE:

ACCELERATE YOUR GAINS WITH THE BRAND-NEW MUSCLE ACTIVATION SETS WARM-UP GUIDE, DEDICATED TO "SWITCHING ON" THE TARGETED MUSCLE SO THAT YOU SUPERCHARGE YOUR WORKOUT AND SET THE STAGE TO GAIN 30 POUNDS OF PURE MUSCLE...THE NATURAL WAY!

Do you want to get the best bang for your workout buck? Do you want to improve a weak body part? Do you want to learn how to activate your muscles more effectively for a better muscle pump and, ultimately, your best body ever?

The Muscle Activation Warm-Up Guide will introduce you to the world of activation sets for more productive workouts, harder muscle contractions, faster gains, and reduced injury risk. Activation sets squeeze the most out of every workout by turning on the right muscles so they fire optimally when you need them. Best of all, activation sets don't take much time, just a few minutes max, so you can easily fit them into your workout. After you start experiencing superior muscle contraction, you'll never attempt another workout without them.

Plus, you'll be added to my B.S.-free VIP newsletter where I debunk the biggest bodybuilding lies and give you my newest muscle and fitness advice to keep you highly motivated, always growing, and ahead of the pack.

JOIN US AND GET INSTANT ACCESS
GetLivingLarge.com/ActivationSets

CONTENTS

PART 5
MASS MECHANICS: UNLOCKING THE PRINCIPLES OF OWNERSHIP, RESPECT & DISADVANTAGES FOR IMMEDIATE GAINS

PART 6
THE ULTIMATE 30-WEEK, ZERO GUESSWORK MUSCLE-BUILDING PROGRAM

PART 7
THE EXERCISE EXECUTION DEMONSTRATION GUIDE: DON'T DO ANOTHER REP WITHOUT THESE MAX CONTRACTION CUES

PART 8
FIVE RITUALS TO RAPID RECOVERY

Contents

INTRODUCTION

> *WARNING!* IF YOU WERE BLESSED WITH GREAT GENES, WANT TO LOOK LIKE A "BODYBUILDING MUTANT," OR IF YOU THINK STEROIDS AND SUPPLEMENTS ARE THE ANSWER, THEN CLOSE THIS BOOK RIGHT NOW. IT'S NOT FOR YOU.

"Scrawny," "Bones," "Toothpick," "Pencil Neck," "String Bean"—I've been called them all. I bet you have too. And if you're like I was, you've searched all the bookstores and scoured the Internet looking for someone to explain to you how to gain weight and build life-changing muscle. You found plenty of information on how to lose weight, but it seems no one wants to help the skinny guy.

Tell friends that you hate being thin, and you're trying to *gain weight,* and they just roll their eyes and tell you you're *lucky.*

Want to know what's worse? No one cares! No one cares that no matter how hard you train, your muscles will not grow as fast as you want them to. No one cares that guys mock you and girls pity you. No one but a skinny guy can understand the disadvantages of your ectomorph physique.

I'm Vince Del Monte, and I am excited that you are reading this book! Why? Because mine is the first book written by an ex-skinny guy specifically for skinny guys like you. My nickname used to be "Skinny Vinny." Now I'm called the "Skinny Guy Savior." I came into this world as a scrawny, awkward pipsqueak. I mean, I had no muscle mass whatsoever. The only thing I wanted was to be big and muscular and not be intimidated by the bigger guys at school.

Adding to my misery, when I got to university, all my roommates were jacked and ripped. I'm talking six-packs, eight-packs, and guns the size of Howitzers! I wanted what they had, but I was a puny runner with a lame social life. I figured I was destined to be "Skinny Vinny" forever.

I started to believe everyone who said, "It's not your fault. You have bad genetics," and, for a while, I gave up the fascination with being muscular, but I still wanted to make the most of the skinny body I was cursed with.

I become a triathlete—a lean and mean swimming, biking, and running machine. I actually got good at it, and I competed at the provincial and national levels. I became the captain of my university squad and even represented my country at the world triathlon championships one year.

But it wasn't everything I wanted.

Just like you, I wanted muscle and respect. Just like you, I wanted to be ripped and feel confident. Just like you, I wanted all the things I figured I could never have.

After four years of university, my athletic eligibility was over, and it was time for me to move into the real world. Like just about everyone else who graduates from an exercise sciences program, I had no

I know too painfully well about your trials and struggles to put on muscle. I know how it feels to walk into the gym where it seems like everyone is growing except you. I know what it's like to go to the beach and wish you didn't have to take your shirt off around cute girls, or to feel intimidated when you walk into a bar or club surrounded by guys who are more muscular than you. I know how annoying it is to not be able to find clothes that reveal a strong and proportioned body or to feel frustrated when you step into a confrontation and you don't have enough respect for yourself to *man up*.

But finding your identity in how many "likes" you get on your shirtless Facebook selfies will suck your soul dry. Freaking out over a missed meal or the next meal, falling in love with the mirror, pushing through injuries that should be rested, revolving the day around me, me, me, leaves you isolated and obsessive.

Don't worry. I'm not promoting any of that crap in here.

This book is about believing in yourself enough to build an empowering and well-proportioned physique that exceeds your body's normal limits and represents you being in control of your life.

> ### *This book is about believing in yourself enough to build an empowering and well-proportioned physique that exceeds your body's normal limits and represents you being in control of your life.*

It's about living large in the gym *and* in life.

When I talk about building life-changing muscle, I mean that along with the big biceps, you develop the self-confidence to approach the lady of your dreams when you see her. That you feel relaxed and at ease in the company of great men. That you become a man of strength and influence around your coworkers, employees, your spouse, children, parents, and friends.

Does having muscle give you all that? No. But going through the process of building it in a natural and sane way does.

Yes, it is possible. You can build the buff body you want without becoming obsessive, working out two hours a day, or spending thousands of dollars on supplements. And you definitely don't need to screw around with steroids.

It doesn't matter if you're a skinny guy who calls himself a "hard-gainer." It doesn't matter if you've been training seriously for six months to a year and have little to show for it. It doesn't matter if you've had some initial success, but your gains have come to a screeching halt. It doesn't matter if you're out of shape. It doesn't matter if you're suffering from "skinny-fat" syndrome. It doesn't matter if you are a complete beginner to weight training, already built and ready to take it to the next level, or making a comeback.

Whatever the case, you have no need to stress because soon you'll learn how I overcame my genetics and built an exceptional physique, and how I've helped more than 150,000 others in 120 different

countries who have bought my programs, and the 750,000+ people who follow me on Facebook and the 300,000 who subscribe to my YouTube channel do the same.

In May 2006, I released my first e-book, *No-Nonsense Muscle Building: Skinny Guy Secrets to Insane Muscle Gain*, and it went on to sell 81,300 copies in 120 countries and became the number-one-selling muscle-building e-book for skinny guys.

Since then I've released numerous digital programs, including *The Live Large Inner Circle, Your Six Pack Quest, Maximize Your Muscle, 21-Day Fast Mass Building, Live Large TV, Stage Shredded Status, 1,000 Rep Muscle, The 7x7 Size & Strength Solution, Hypertrophy MAX, Get Juiced, 1-on-1 High Level Physique & Performance Coaching, The Vanity Specialization Programs, No-Nonsense Muscle Building 2.0*, and *Maximize Your Muscle 2.0*.

As I write this, my first e-book is almost ten years old. That's like a million years in "Internet time."

I've learned a lot since then, and I've added a ton of upgrades based on new science that wasn't available in 2006. Every claim I make and every recommendation I give is backed by the latest and best research. I've traveled the world speaking to today's top experts. I've hired the best coaches. I've found the sources with the best research. I've tested the information on my own physique as well as the people I coach, so you don't have to.

This book isn't like anything else I've ever released. I've condensed the best information I've found to date and put it in a format to give you only usable content, with no fat—nothing but meat. This is a book you can bring anywhere you want and open it at any point to pull out muscle-building advice you can benefit from immediately.

I wrote this book because I want to give the muscle-building community an easy-to-read, portable resource where you can find the information you want fast, when you need it. It has a detailed table of contents, so you can look up the information you need, and get right to it. You don't have to wade through pages and pages of fluff to find the one point you need to clarify or the one exercise you want to try next.

The goal of this book is simple: to help you pack on 30 pounds of life-changing muscle in the next 30 weeks . . . the natural way. It's a big promise, and it's doable . . . but it won't be easy. (If you've already gained more than 30 pounds of rock-solid muscle since you began lifting, don't expect another 30 pounds from this book, but do expect some extraordinary results.)

Some of the highlights include a brand-new 30-week step-by-step three-phase program based on DTS Training—the most scientific, most strategic, and simplest way to build life-changing muscle. It includes a complete set of simple, no-nonsense meal plans that eliminate all the nutritional guesswork. It tells you the only four supplements to consider if you desire to optimize your results.

As for the workouts, I won't just show you what to do in the gym but how to do it. This is the first and only book that teaches you *what to think* when moving a weight from point A to point B, along with the most biomechanically effective cues.

I'll expose how the bodybuilding industry has been scamming you out of your time and money, so you'll no longer be a casualty of misinformation, and you will learn the bottom-line truth about gaining weight and building lean muscle the no-nonsense way.

By purchasing this book, you've put your trust in me as your coach. I know you're busy and a lot of things are fighting for your attention. The most valuable things I can ask from you are your time and attention. I respect that above anything else, and I promise not to waste it. I understand that, even though there is no one out there purely dedicated to the skinny guy like I am, there are a ton of muscular dudes who could teach you a thing or two about building your body, so I'm honored that you've decided to give me your attention and spend your time with me. Here's how this book is different than any other muscle and fitness book you have read:

1. Everything Is Backed by Science

There was a period when I was uploading so much content that people started to challenge the quality. I started hearing people call me a "bro-scientist" online.

At first, I wrote them off as "haters," but as I did some further research, I realized I hadn't done my due diligence, and I was doing my audience a disservice. I have some of my biggest critics to thank for inspiring me to go to a "quality vs. quantity" model when it comes to sharing content on my blog, Facebook page, newsletter, and YouTube channel.

I wrote this book with the most evidence-based science guys in mind. I want them to be able to read this book and say, "This is really good."

Any claim I make is backed with a reference, so you can be sure nothing I am saying is simply my opinion or pulled out of my rear.

2. Everything Is Backed by Gains

Based on what I said above, you may wonder if I only follow the science. Absolutely not. Effective bodybuilding involves art and science, but frankly, it is more of an art. Don't blindly conform everything you do to the latest study because scientific conclusions do not always meet the needs of the individual. I have adopted or discarded all of my approaches based on a combination of personal experience, clients' experiences, and the scientific data available. Use the science as a starting point, but then use your intuition and modify the program based on what works for you. Don't be afraid to conduct your own personal experiments. Test, tweak, and optimize. You don't need a study to justify every single action. All that matters is that you take action every day, keep what works for you, and throw away what doesn't.

3. I Don't Just Teach This Stuff, I Live and Breathe It

There are a ton of people teaching muscle, fitness, and fat loss whom I call "me-too experts." That means they are not saying anything different or bringing anything new. They are repackaging the same old material you've heard a million times already in a sexier way or with a new hook. And they don't always practice what they teach. They have a lukewarm passion for fitness but a burning passion for profits and cashing in on people's fears and insecurities. I'm here to do something about that. My goal is to be your go-to resource when it comes to building muscle without the foolishness or fearmongering. If someone pulled the plug on the Internet tomorrow, you would still find me in the gym grinding away.

4. I Don't Just Learn from the Internet; I Rub Shoulders with Real Experts

Warning: the majority of the information you read online is bad information. If you're constantly adopting your strategies from things you learned from headlines and fitness marketing, you'll always struggle. I want to help you avoid "shiny object syndrome" and keep you focused on easy-to-understand and quick-to-implement advice that works.

5. I Cut Straight to the Chase . . . No-Nonsense Style

I wanted to write a book that gives you advice you can follow right now and see a result right after you apply it. I included the word "no-nonsense" in the subtitle of my book, so I'd have to live up to it. A fitness book should contain clear marching orders with no fluff. It should inspire and motivate. It should help you believe in your ability. It should be easy to toss in your gym bag and bring with you to workouts.

So, here's to your new ripped and muscular physique and becoming the next *Biggest Gainer*!

Train HARD, train SMARTER, build FASTER, and, after 30 weeks, send me your before-and-after photos, so I can celebrate with you, and I would be honored to share your story on my social media platforms.

Vince DelMonte

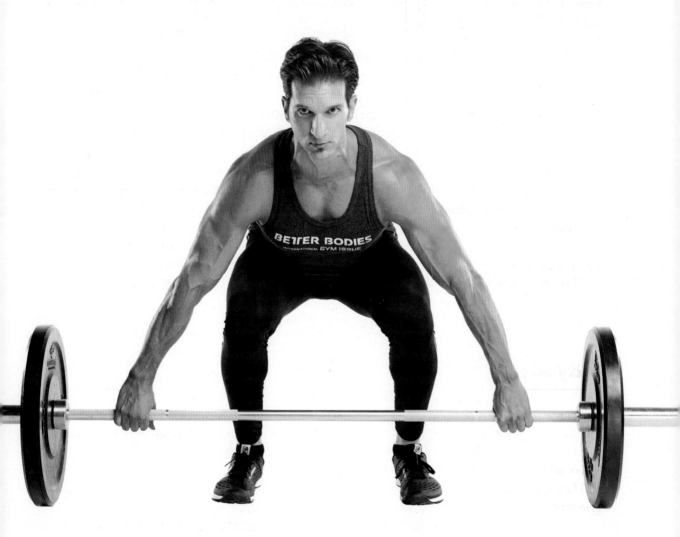

"Nothing in business or life is more expensive than bad information."
—GARY HALBERT

PART 1
Muscle Misinformation: The Five Muscle-Building Enemies You Must Avoid

The muscle and fitness industry is full of more lies, myths, and total B.S. than nearly any industry on the planet. Some good information is getting through, but in most magazines, social media venues, and mainstream media, the information is flat-out wrong.

While there are plenty of charlatans and scammers out there, I don't believe the majority of fitness "gurus" are intentionally lying. They are repeating lies they believe to be true. Overwhelmed with information overload, the fitness industry is becoming a case of the blind following the blind.

My duty and mission is to bust industry myths and deliver to you the most direct and efficient way to build muscle—without the nonsense or foolishness.

Let's get started.

Naysayers—How to Deal with Them

When I started bodybuilding, my father caught me checking myself out in the mirror, admiring my newfound muscles while taking mental "selfies," and he questioned me, "What are you doing? Are you in love with yourself? What is this sport?"

He walked away shaking his head. I felt embarrassed.

I love my father. I trust him. I respect him, and he has always encouraged me. If I'd been inclined to give up on my goal due to anyone's opinion, my father's would have been it.

Rather than interpret his skepticism as a reason to stop, I used it to remind myself that my building muscle needed to have a bigger purpose than just looking good. I took the gift and kept going.

Naysayers come in many forms, and often there's a grain of truth in what they say. Your job is to take the useful part of the message and discard the rest.

Some naysayers are just ignorant. Do not believe anyone who tells you that you can only have an average body. Average results come out of average knowledge and average effort. They are not destiny.

To add 30 pounds of muscle you must first obtain your own 100 percent commitment. Do not allow naysayers in any form to dissuade you. Instead, turn their doubt into your determination. Let their ignorance ignite your passion. Turn their ridicule into your resolve.

Know in your heart that you are doing the right things. Do not waste any energy arguing or trying to convince. The results show soon enough. Let your muscular body do the talking. When naysayers see the change in you, they will either shut up or tell everyone they always knew you could do it.

Bodybuilding Magazines—Why I Tossed Mine in the Garbage

Fashion magazines exist to sell clothes and makeup. Advertisers hire gorgeous models, airbrush the photos so they look flawless, and then use the perfected images to sell their wares. Bodybuilding magazines are similar in that they exist to sell supplements. Advertisers use photographs of shredded models with huge muscles, and every month they tell you that your dream body is locked up inside some liquid, powder, or pill.

Don't buy it. Aside from the very few exceptions that I'll share with you, every new supplement is made with the same crap that the last supplement had. If a bodybuilding magazine spent all two hundred pages of one issue teaching you how to properly eat and weight train, then you wouldn't have the desire to buy *any* supplements. Supplement sellers would stop buying ad space, and the magazine would be out of business.

And that's just what it is—a business. While they inspire millions, bodybuilding magazines also mislead millions. They aren't going to tell you the truth—that drugs combined with exceptional genetics are responsible for these guys' massive size. Just like the fashion model will say, "It's the mascara," the featured hulks will claim their results came from supplements because they're being paid to promote them.

Most of the routines recommended in these magazines would kill an adult gorilla. The workouts involve so much volume, even if you can do them for a while, it's not sustainable. It's like asking a beginning runner to sprint a marathon, five times a week. If you're not taking steroids, the advice in these articles will cause overtraining, injuries, or illness, and lots of wasted time, and you should avoid them.

Personal Trainers Who Are More About Sales Than Size

You shouldn't pump iron without expert guidance, but finding a good trainer can be a real challenge. In the fitness world, it's pretty easy to become an "overnight expert"—take your shirt off, show your abs, start a YouTube channel, and you're in business. It's one thing to change your own physique, but helping others requires another skill-set. The best trainers have one aim—and it's not to cause you the most pain, make you sore, or chew your ear off and waste your time. It *is* to get you to your goal optimally and safely with nonstop progress.

As of this writing, no state agency sets standards for, regulates, or monitors personal trainers. Some trainers get "certified" by just taking a written test online, but even a degree in exercise physiology does not mean the trainer knows how to help you gain size. Most teach exercise and give nutrition advice designed to help the general public improve overall fitness. They do not deliver specialized knowledge on how to gain massive amounts of muscle.

Working for a gym or having years of experience doesn't guarantee your trainer knows what he's doing either. Most gyms survive not on memberships but by selling personal training packages, and a lot of them hire novice trainers to do it. If you go to your local big-box gym and look, you're more likely to meet a great salesperson than a kick-ass trainer.

Know what to look for and which questions to ask. Do a demo session or two. Ask about the last certification or seminar they invested in. Ask who mentors them. Make sure the trainer has his or her own coach and stays up-to-date on the latest science. I instantly disqualify potential trainers who don't have their own coach. It sounds harsh, but this one rule will help you rule out average trainers.

Only keep a trainer who comes to the session with the attitude that for every minute that he's not delivering value, that's a dollar back to you. If they show up 15 minutes late, that should be a $15 discount on the session. If they're rambling about nothing for 10 minutes, that's $10 off!

Look for someone with a solid track record who has helped others achieve the results you want. Ask to see their success stories. Look at or talk to their other clients. If your prospective mentor doesn't have a track record of success helping people achieve goals identical to yours, then you've dodged a bullet. Move on.

"Superhumans" and the Juiced-Up Bodybuilder

Eight-time Mr. Olympia champion Jay Cutler bench-pressed 315 pounds the first time he lifted weights.[1] Rumor has it that Arnold ripped out his own umbilical cord. Some people were born to develop massive size and strength. If at age sixteen you looked like Arnold Schwarzenegger when he was sixteen, you wouldn't need this book to gain size. The genetically gifted can lift more. They don't get as sore. They recover faster. So, yeah, they have an unfair advantage.

For you to try to follow their regimen to get their results is ridiculous. It's like a poor man taking wealth-building advice from a guy who inherited a fortune. Even though he has the money, he doesn't know how to go from broke to wealthy. His methods don't apply.

The juiced-up bodybuilder is also your enemy, and if he's lying about taking steroids, it's worse. When you follow the advice of these "fake naturals" or "fake nattys" and fail to get great results, it can strip you of your motivation. Problem is, almost everyone who takes steroids hides it, making you believe it's the "hard training," "clean diet," and "new breakthrough program" that forced that muscle growth. "B.S.," I say. If a fitness guru is taking steroids, he should at least be honest about it so people can see the whole picture.

Gizmos and Gadgets

The next time you find yourself sitting on the couch late at night watching an infomercial for fitness equipment or a quick-fix nutritional product, drop and give me 20 pushups—one-handed—while repeating, "I'm not a sucker . . . I'm not a sucker . . ." That ought to wake you up out of your stupor before you get your credit card and buy a $1,000 coatrack. Whether or not it's you, I bet you know someone with a massive "fitness" contraption that has become the world's most expensive clothesline, because thousands of people buy this crap.

A good sign of how well a product is selling is how long the ads run.[2] No advertiser would keep running an ad unless it sold *a lot* of product. Good marketing can get people to buy all kinds of things, but let's face it, if you think any fitness model built his body using a vibrating dumbbell, you're dreaming. These guys got buff with hours in the gym and hard work, so keep your ass off the couch and your hand off the remote. You can build mega muscle mass without spending a ton of money on equipment or supplements. If you have some money to put into this quest, spend it on high-quality food, a decent gym membership, and a solid coach.

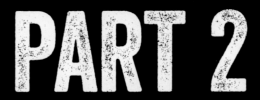

PART 2

How to Lose the Top Five B.S. Excuses for Not Gaining Muscle

So many people ask me how to build muscle, and I tell them—I belong to a gym, eat healthy, stay consistent, educate myself, and take a few select supplements. Next they unload an earful of excuses, excuses, excuses. I am so sick and tired of hearing excuses! I have zero sympathy for people who make excuses. All it means is they haven't taken responsibility for their lives.

Your life today is the result of choices you made before. You can take responsibility for everything you have in life, or you can choose to blame others and outside forces. I have found that the results you achieve in and out of the gym rarely exceed your willingness to stop making excuses and start taking personal responsibility for everything you have, do, and are at this moment and every moment to come. Next up are the typical excuses and how to overcome them.

> *Your life today is the result of choices you made before.*
> *You can take responsibility for everything you have in life,*
> *or you can choose to blame others and outside forces.*

Cut the "I Don't Have Great Genetics" Crap

Most people think they are limited by their genetic potential. Really, you're limited by your *lifestyle potential*. You don't need great genetics. You do need to train hard, eat right, be consistent, and excel in all the lifestyle areas you *can* control.

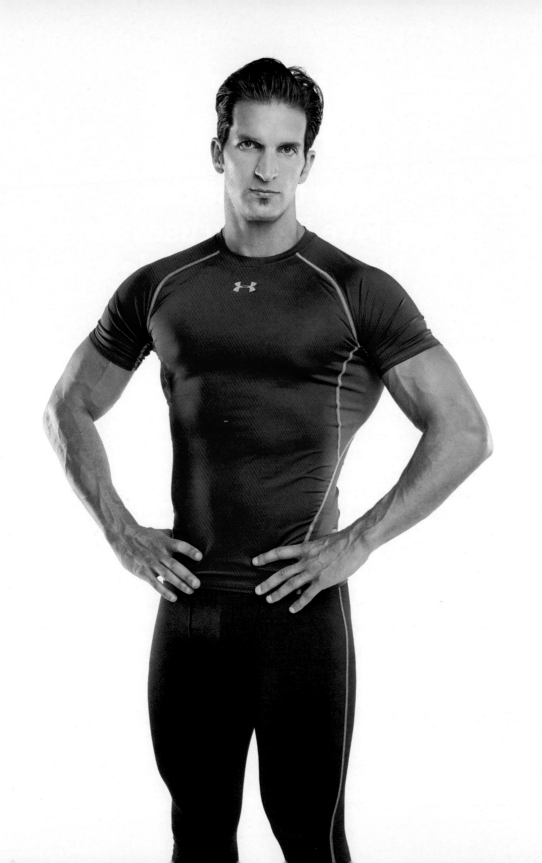

Your genes don't determine what you can or can't do. They express how your body responds to what you do. I've helped scores of men and women who thought they were genetically destined to be skinny or fat achieve their goals just by fixing a few things they were doing wrong.

It's true that guys with great genetics can afford to make more mistakes in training and nutrition strategies, and they may still get bigger faster than most.

> ### *Your genes don't determine what you can or can't do.*
> ### *They express how your body responds to what you do.*

If you build muscle a little slower, the added time it takes to get there is irrelevant. It might take one guy one year and take you two years. Big deal.

If you're afraid you can't build the body you want and maintain it, throw those fears out. The only people who can't build muscle have a terminal disease.

If, like me, you were born with the genetics to be a skinny guy, you're not doomed to remain skinny. But you need to be more scientific and strategic. I'm going to teach you to do what's necessary. Nothing more. Nothing less.

One more thing I want you to experience: satisfaction. Nothing is more satisfying than overcoming a legitimate obstacle and reaching your goal. Your transformation will inspire others, so the next skinny guy will say, "Holy cow, he did it! Why can't I?"

(Remember, this book is about building life-changing muscle, not just self-serving muscle.)

Quit Saying, "I Don't Have Enough Money"

I've never heard anyone complain about putting in a lot of money when they're getting a big return on investment, have you?

The top three investments I've made have gone to food, mentoring, and a great MAT™ (Muscle Activation Technique) therapist, and I've received exponential returns—in my body and in my business. You don't have to be a fitness expert to benefit from having a great physique. *TIME* magazine reported in June 2012 a study by the *Journal of Labor Research* that found employees who exercise earn 9 percent more than those who don't.

Invest in your weakest link. Eating organic is healthier, but it won't have a "game-changing" impact on your results, so if you want to be frugal, maybe you'll buy conventional and wash your produce a little more thoroughly. Maybe your weakest link is in the gym. If you don't train with enough intensity or you are having trouble finding a workout partner who is as committed as you, invest in a trainer.

Supplements—the few that work—only have a marginal impact, maybe a 10 percent improvement, in your results, so hold off on most of those for now. Later, I'll show you the four supplements that you can't go without.

For the next 30 weeks, I'm asking you to prioritize your finances toward this goal. You don't need to spend a ton of money, but if you're willing to invest some, you will see more gains.

Drop the "I Don't Have a Lot of Time" Speech

If you think you don't have any time, then I'm not sure why you're reading this book. Put the book down and go make up your mind about what your priorities are. If you're not ready to show up, I can't help you. No one can help you. You're beyond help. If you don't have time now, you never will. Life gets faster, busier. Start with the time you do have. You don't need a lot.

The first time I trained with one of my mentors, I ended up puking in the bathroom after six sets of body weight split squats. It took nine minutes. I was used to pumping out a couple dozen "junk sets" for an hour and a half, but he raised the intensity so high that after the first few sets, I was done. I didn't need to do anymore. I saw black spots for days.

If you're training a lot but not intensely, you might even need to make your workouts shorter. Most people aren't *investing* time in the gym. They are spending it. Wasting it. Most guys try to work out six days a week with 18 to 24 sets per workout (inspired by the misleading "muscle & fiction" magazines). You don't need that many sets. You didn't earn it. Time in the gym has to be earned. Volume has to be earned. Learn to get the most out of one set, then add more sets. Don't add more volume *until you've earned the need for more*. Get the most out of the least amount of effort. Eliminate junk sets. Pare down to the "minimum effective dose" of workout time. Get in. Get it done. Get out. The solution to building 30 pounds of muscle in 30 weeks is focused intense effort in the moment—making each rep, each set, each workout matter.

If you're training for zero minutes a week right now, even five minutes will help. Do three killer sets in five minutes, and you will grow.

No More "I'm Too _____" (Insert Your Limiting Belief Here)

Everyone has some B.S. story that they pull out as an excuse of why they can't reach their goals. I had the limiting belief that I always blow my diet when I go on a trip. Thinking that way, I was giving myself permission to get off course, and I became my own worst enemy. I shared my frustrations with others who used the same excuse. "Oh, yeah, me too!" they would say, and that only reinforced my belief that it was beyond my control.

It wasn't until I met a guy who traveled as much as I did, who went to as many five-star hotels and restaurants, but was absolutely shredded. He didn't have any trouble staying lean and continuing to make gains.

"What do you do?" I asked.

"I don't drink booze, and I avoid appetizers and dessert," he said.

"Huh? I can do that. I can cut the dessert!" I thought. And so I did, and I saw that I too could come home from a trip looking just as good as when I left.

I changed my story about what's possible, tried a new strategy, and the results changed my belief!

> ### *Find the areas where you think you're being held back by some mysterious power. Realize these are the areas where you need a better story and a better strategy.*

For you, no whining and no wallowing. Find the areas where you think you're being held back by some mysterious power. Realize these are the areas where you need a better story and a better strategy. Whatever your limiting story is, make up an empowering one to replace it. Wherever you use a faulty strategy, get a new one.

Establish new patterns and habits. Hang out with people who have raised their standards and commitment to the level that's required to get the results you want. Whenever I go out with these friends, I don't even worry about willpower, because I know they're not ordering.

> *"The mind is the limit. As long as the mind can envision the fact you can do something, you can do it."*
> **—ARNOLD SCHWARZENEGGER**

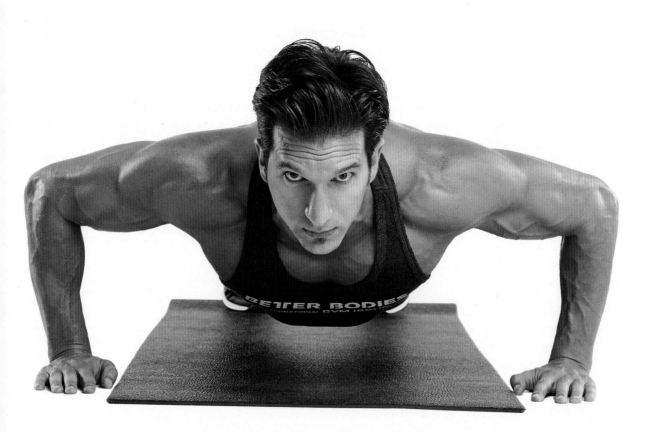

PART 3

Use Your Brain to Add Brawn: Seven Key Mind-Set Strategies

Your muscle-building success is all in your head. When you compare good physiques to great physiques, mind-set is the difference maker. Building a better body isn't about what your muscles can do; it's what your mind believes is possible and having the right strategies to guide your belief. Anyone who has trained consistently hard with focus, desire, and discipline knows that the brain will beg you to drop the weight and call it a day long before your muscles are truly finished.

> *Building a better body isn't about what your muscles can do; it's what your mind believes is possible and having the right strategies to guide your belief.*

To get the best results with this challenging 30-week program, go into each set with a certainty that you have what it takes to move the weight and hit the number of reps you need to crush.

While you may conceptually buy into the idea of unwavering conviction, it helps to have a set of strategies that bring out the best in you, and that's what we're going to cover next.

Set Goals in HD

A lot of guys say they know what their goals are, but really, they only have a vague sense. To actually reach a big goal, you need to set it in HD.

A high-def goal has four components: it's specific, realistic, measurable, and has a due date. Let's look at each one.

Specific: If you start out saying, "I want to gain a lot of muscle," that is not specific enough. The key to unlocking your motivation is to state exactly what you plan to achieve. "I will gain 30 pounds of muscle in the next six months."

Realistic: Notice I didn't suggest you make goals too pie-in-the-sky. Don't say you'll take six months to "go from 150-pounds to 250-pounds and ripped." If a goal is too high, you do yourself a disservice. Make a goal that forces you to stretch your limits, but also is attainable within the designated timeframe.

Measurable: CEOs of billion-dollar companies know that what gets measured gets managed and what gets managed gets multiplied. Many of the world's top CEOs got where they are because they measure everything—profits, costs, markets, productivity, and on and on. The same rules apply here. Set goals you can measure—size gains, body fat percentage, target weight, or whatever ties to your desired outcome, then state the number(s) you want and track your progress, so you can course-correct when you need to.

Due Date: I bet you never took a course where the teacher said the final would be given "at some point." All the important things in life have a due date, because without one, a lot of important things would not get done. Paying bills and taxes, planning a wedding, raising money for a specific event—all of these have dates by which they must get done, or there will be consequences. The same is true with your fitness goals. Set a deadline to reach your goal, and define some consequences. Decide what happens if you don't.

Shrink the Change

One meal at a time, one workout at a time, one day at a time. That's all it takes. If you shrink the change down to these small increments and daily actions, you'll grow faster, and in 30 weeks, you'll achieve your absolute best body so far.

When you're at the beginning, don't obsess about what's going to happen in the middle, because the middle will look different when you get there. It's like when you're traveling, you can look at a map, but you don't know for sure what that road will look like until you're driving on it.

Have a sense of urgency to do what's most important right now. If you're reading this before you go to bed, and you haven't prepared your meals for tomorrow, close the book, go to the kitchen, and prep your meals. Once you've done that, make sure your next workout is printed out, your training partner knows what time to meet, and that you know exactly what you're going to do when you get to the gym.

Don't worry today about a strong finish six or seven months from now. You have no business even worrying about next week! Don't try to anticipate every turn on the road. That's impossible. Focus on what is right in front of you. All you need to know is the very next thing you need to do, and then *do it*. Just focus on taking each step one at a time, and make today the best day ever.

Focus on what is right in front of you.
All you need to know is the very next thing
you need to do, and then do it.

Focus on Habits, Not Outcomes

Guys with great bodies built great habits over an extended period of time.

Instead of comparing yourself to others, obsessing over factors you can't control, or focusing too much on the desired result, focus on the daily habits that will achieve that result—meal preparation, workout scheduling, training intensely, grocery shopping, getting sufficient sleep, listening to your coach, and social support and accountability with like-minded trainees. I know some of this information isn't very sexy, but it's always the nonsexy stuff that gets the best results.

A good friend of mine, John Berardi, taught me to implement habits that provide the greatest physical benefit with the least psychological resistance. Develop the habit of waking up and having a cup of water with lemon to help cleanse your body and hydrate. Or start taking fish oils. How hard is it to take two pills every day? But that's going to start helping your body utilize fats and carbs better. Or build the habit of getting five to ten servings of veggies every day, and after a month it has a huge impact on your body's ability to recover.

Habits stack on top of each other. As you develop more good habits, you'll see a cumulative effect. If you can build one new habit a month that helps you grow, just imagine where you'll be a year from now with twelve new muscle-building habits.

Slow Equals Fast

If you think you're going to transform your body (I mean dramatically) in two to four weeks, slap yourself and wake up!

Although rapid muscle growth is possible at the very beginning for novice lifters, serious muscle building is a long and tedious process.

Be patient. It takes six to twelve months to gain your first 30 to 40 pounds of lean mass. If you try to grow too fast, putting yourself through a killer workout your first night at the gym, cutting your calories to 1,000 a day and going into starvation mode, and trying out six new supplements at once, you'll end up sore, sick, and broke—if you're lucky. If you're not lucky, you'll also end up injured.

Successful people are task completers. They are quick to commit and slow to change their minds. They realize that anything worth having comes with a price, and they are willing to pay it. They pick a solid plan and stick to it until they reach the goal, making slight adjustments as needed along the way.

Focus on making consistent and incremental improvements over time, and you'll be happy with your results.

View Weaknesses as Strengths

I'm an open book when it comes to how I built my online fitness business. If people ask me for advice, I share what I know. Many years ago, someone tried to tell me that was a weakness. "You've got to hold your cards closer to your chest, man. You reveal way too much."

Look at everything as a positive. Even your perceived weaknesses are helping you right now.

For a little while, I listened to him, and I stayed quiet. But I stopped seeing the reciprocation from others. I wasn't putting out as much goodwill, so I got less in return. I realized then that my so-called "weakness" of sharing my best business practices was really a strength. This holds true in the gym. For example, one positive of being skinny is that it's harder for you to gain fat.

Look at everything as a positive. Even your perceived weaknesses are helping you right now.

I don't care that I'm not the biggest guy, or the strongest, or the most articulate. I might view all this as a weakness in building my online business, but I don't. My physique is attainable. It's realistic. That makes me relatable, and that's a strength I play to. I don't have extraordinary genetics, yet I make the most of what I do have, and that has allowed me to inspire hundreds of thousands of guys and gals to strive to be their best.

What do I care if some guy looks at me and says, "That guy's not even big. He's a joke"? Real, regular, everyday people can look at me and say, "He's real. I could achieve that. I want to learn more from this guy."

Right now, write down the top ten weaknesses you think are holding you back, and transform them into ten reasons to succeed.

Let Go of "I Know"

My good friend Peter, a brilliant man who's no longer with us, taught me an important lesson about "I know." He drew a little circle on a whiteboard and put a dot in the middle, pointed to it, and said, "This is me in the middle here."

*The only way to really know whether anything is true
is to take what you've learned and create a result.*

Then he shaded in the rest of the circle. "This is everything I know within the circle. And then, when I learn something that I didn't know..." He drew another circle on the outside of the circle. "I realized that there's a whole other circle that's surrounding the first circle, new information, and a whole bunch of stuff I didn't know!"

He explained that the more we learn within each circle, there's another circle beyond that, and in the end, "The more you learn, the more you realize how little you know."

Very often, we think we "know" something because we've heard it said so much. But the only way to really know whether anything is true is to take what you've learned and create a result.

You might look at some of the strategies here and say, "I knew that." But there's a big difference between *knowing* what to do and actually *doing* it. So to be frank, if you don't have new muscle mass or strength to show for the knowledge, you don't really know it. You don't know anything until you have something to show for it.

Belief Is Better Than Steroids

Whatever you want to achieve, believe you can do it, and you will. Act "as if" you already have the 30 pounds of muscle. Carry yourself with the same confidence. Think about your day from that perspective. Make decisions as the guy who *already has* bulging muscles and six-pack abs, and you will become him.

This applies outside the gym as well. Before I met my wife, I dated this girl I liked a lot. I swore she was The One, but she dumped me after three weeks. I never forgot her because of what she said: "Look at it as a positive. God never sticks you with second best. If you liked me, just imagine how amazing the woman you're going to marry is!"

I believed what she told me was true. I took that belief with me into every relationship I had after that, and I viewed every breakup as a positive.

I later dated one girl for a year and a half. I thought she was The One, too, and when that ended, I thought, "Wow! I wonder what the next one is going to be like?"

My belief kept me going with a positive mind-set all the way up to the day I met my wife. I knew as soon as I met Flavia that she *really was* The One. We were engaged within six months, married six months after that and at the time of this writing, we have a little girl and a baby boy.

Keep your belief alive. No matter what you want, it will power you towards your goal with more strength and speed than even the world's most advanced steroids could . . . and no bad side effects.

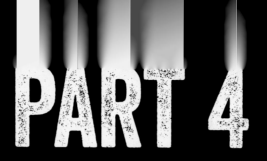

PART 4

Five Essential Training Principles to Gain Your First 30 Pounds of Pure Muscle

Ask any good coach about a complex problem, and the first response you're likely to get is, "It depends."

As much as it may seem like a boring, wishy-washy half-answer, this is the best answer because "it depends…" acknowledges that it's best to know more about the situation and the context of the question before giving definitive advice. The good news is that gaining your first 30 pounds of muscle is *not a complex problem*. Until you gain your first 30 pounds of muscle, you don't deserve to ask questions that require an "it depends" answer.

I have done it and hundreds of my top clients have done it, and because this book is based on the no-nonsense strategy of achieving that goal, we will start with the five essential training principles where *not one factor* falls into the realm of "it depends."

If you try out this program and you're not gaining muscle, come back to these five principles.

Get Lean to Get Big

If you stand shirtless in front of the mirror, and you can't see a four-pack, you're suffering from the dreaded "Skinny Fat Syndrome." The best advice I can give you is to *get lean first*. I know you might be feeling impatient and want to go right into building mass, but starting off lean will prime your body for rapid muscle gains and fuel your mental drive. If you're starting out lean already, you've got a hormonal advantage[3] and can move right into building mass.

The old-school bodybuilder model of an initial six to twelve-month "bulk up" phase where you eat tremendous amounts of food (and put on a bit of muscle and mostly fat) followed by a three to four-

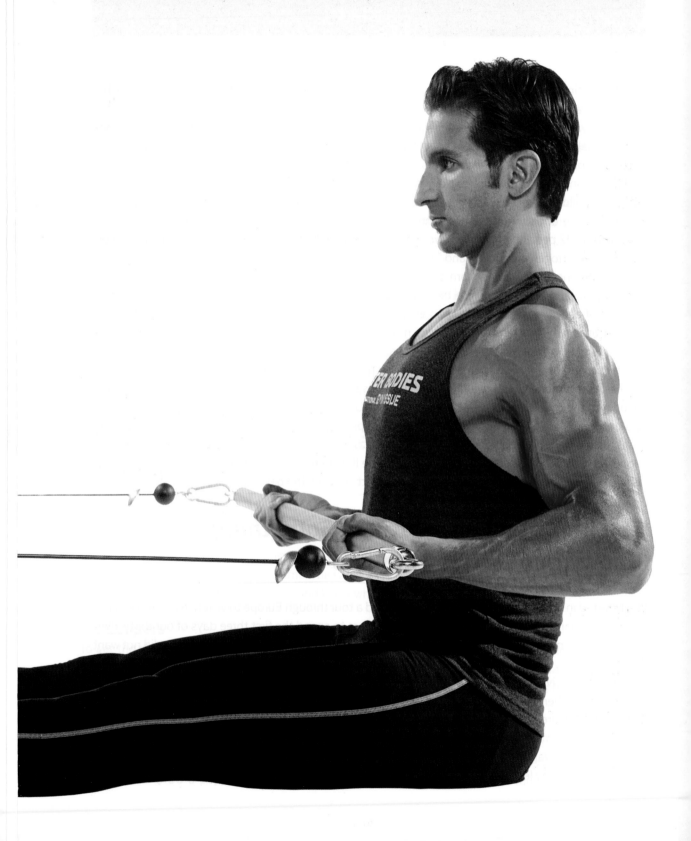

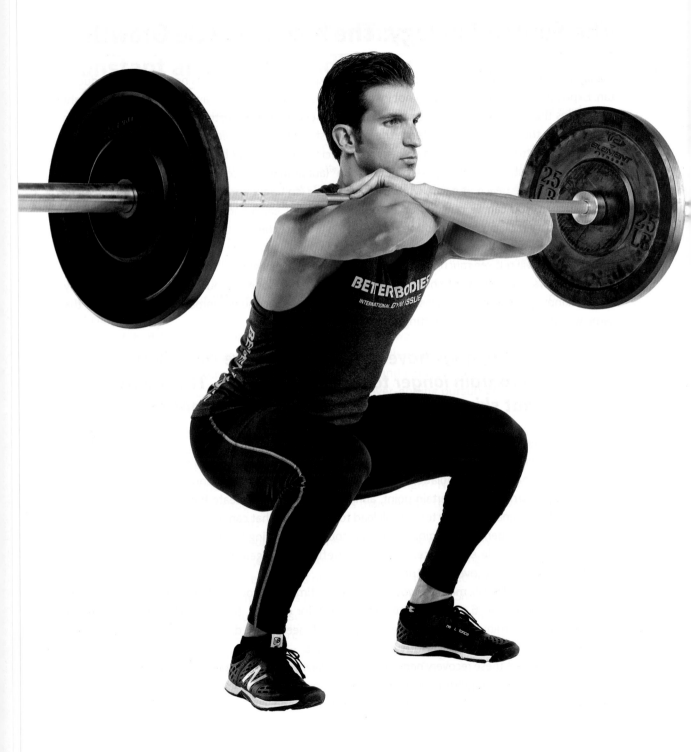

PART 5

Mass Mechanics: Unlocking the Principles of Ownership, Respect & Disadvantages for Immediate Gains

Want to know the number-one reason you struggle to build muscle?

It's not what you think. It has nothing to do with your diet, supplements, workout program, exercise selection, or failing to apply progressive overload. While those are critical aspects to muscle growth, none of these is the number-one reason you can't build muscle. And it's not genetics either. In my opinion, nine times out of ten, it's *ineffective movement*, otherwise known as crappy lifting technique.

Most people in the gym, even guys with great physiques, have never been taught how to move. The goal is to contract the muscle you intend to grow. Most guys go to the gym and swing weights around hoping their muscles will "catch" some contractions, but due to poor movement patterns they often experience contractions in the wrong muscle groups.

The fitness industry is missing the boat on optimal movement. The majority of "gurus" and personal trainers simply have you smash the muscle into oblivion by throwing at it every exercise and intensity technique known to man, hoping to trigger some growth. This is a surefire way to destroy your joints and keep your muscles weak and small (and eventually injured). You've probably tried that approach, which is why you're here now. You're looking for something better and smarter.

Did you know your body doesn't want to build muscle? Not a single ounce more than it needs. Muscle is expensive. It takes a lot of calories to feed and keep it. Your body evolved to be fast and efficient, so it can respond to danger and survive on limited food if necessary.[18]

Your body has zero interest in gaining 30 pounds of muscle over the next 30 weeks, so you need to be prepared to make your body do what you want it to do, not what it wants to do.

The second you pick up a challenging weight, your body is looking for strategies to make that action as efficient and easy as possible because it has no idea how long you're going to need to meet that challenge. Your body will immediately recruit your strongest, most appropriate muscle groups, and when those get tired, it seeks the next best available muscle groups. Essentially, your body is looking for a way to disperse the load you're attempting to lift through as many muscles groups as possible so it can achieve the path of least resistance.

Your body has zero interest in gaining 30 pounds of muscle over the next 30 weeks, so you need to be prepared to make your body do what you want it to do, not what it wants to do.

Let's say you desire a crazy-looking V-tapered back. Even if you're doing the "best back exercises" prescribed by experts, your body has zero idea that you're doing a "back exercise" and will find a way to dump tension into stronger surrounding muscles that pick up the load unless you *teach and train* it to selectively recruit and isolate the back muscles you want to target.

All the "progressive overload" techniques in the world don't mean squat if your exercise execution lacks precision. When your ego dictates how much you lift, your strong muscles get stronger (and more developed), and your weak muscles get weaker (and stay underdeveloped), leaving you with an unbalanced physique.

The good news is that you can break crappy movement patterns by learning my Mass Mechanics Execution Principles—the blueprint to build your muscles as big as you desire.

This information is simple to apply, but you won't find it floating around freely. The only place I've seen it taught is where I learned it, in physical therapist and internationally renowned biomechanics expert Tom Purvis' advanced exercise mechanics personal training course RTS123.com.

My view of exercise completely changed when I took his course. I learned muscles respond to tension and torque. Muscles do not know weight. You must learn how to get your "mind inside the muscle" to maximize tension[19] in muscles you selectively recruit throughout every single inch of the rep. No matter how much weight you put on the bar, no matter what diet you're on, no matter which supplements you take, you will never pack on the kind of mass you desire until you learn how to do this.

Next up, you'll learn the exercise execution principles that will *instantly* unlock new massive growth, so you can see for yourself that there is no such thing as a "weak body part"—just a poorly trained one.

*All the "progressive overload" techniques
in the world don't mean squat if your exercise
execution lacks precision. When your ego
dictates how much you lift, your strong
muscles get stronger (and more developed),
and your weak muscles get weaker (and stay
underdeveloped), leaving you with
an unbalanced physique.*

Mass Mechanics Principle #1: The Principle of Ownership

The number-one component of muscle growth is *time under tension* which comes down to *owning the weight.* You maintain complete control of the tension on the intended muscle from start to finish.

This principle is of the highest importance to muscle growth potential to the point that beginners who learn to maintain control of the muscle tension all the way through the range of motion can have an advantage over advanced lifters who have years of bad movement habits to break and undo.

To use the principle of ownership properly, you must create the greatest challenge possible (maximal tension) for the muscle. The more neuromuscular connection you can generate in the working muscle, the higher the growth potential.

*For muscle growth, if you can't control it,
you can't challenge it, and if you can't challenge it,
you can't grow it.*

To do this, first learn to engage the working muscle throughout the full range of motion (ROM). It's easy to control the midrange, but you're leaving a ton of gains on the table if you don't own every single inch of the movement path, which includes both extremes of the range (the shortened and lengthened positions). It's at the extremes of the ROM where you are the weakest, and anywhere you're weak there is opportunity for growth.

For muscle growth, if you can't control it, you can't challenge it, and if you can't challenge it, you can't grow it.[20]

Want to know whether you own the weight? Imagine doing a squat and during the movement I yell, "STOP!" Would you be able to go into an isometric hold (no movement) at any point of the range? Most importantly, would you be able to hold it at the bottom, where the weight feels the heaviest? If you can, you own that weight. If you can't, it means the weight is controlling you, and you're less likely to see the growth you want and more likely to get injured.

By using these key concepts, you can activate untapped muscle fibers at the extreme ends of the range to build new muscle and take your physique to the next level.

Key Concepts To Apply & Goals To Think About During Your Set

- *"Initiate with the working muscle."* Top bodybuilding coach Ben Pakulski brought this cue to the muscle and fitness world. It reminds you to create tension *before* you start moving. You'll know you're doing this properly if you initiate each movement without using momentum. Instead of swinging the weight like you're in a circus act, to get the weight moving, *contract against the resistance*. Perform this same practice over and over to train your muscles to optimize time under tension.
- *"Beat the weight 1 pound at a time as you lift"* and *"Let the weight beat you 1 pound at a time as you lower."* Think about that for a moment. The muscle should feel every single pound of tension from the beginning of the movement to the very end. This cue reminds you to slow down. If you perform each repetition too fast, it's hard to keep the tension on the targeted muscle. Instead, the tension gets dumped into the joints, which leads to aches, pains, and injuries.
- *"Squeeze the weight, don't swing it."* Momentum is the adversary of gains. If you swing the weight, you can't own it. Aim to squeeze out every single rep using the targeted muscle. You'll know you're doing it right if your muscles are burning like crazy and even begin to cramp. Make every effort to squeeze the weight through your full range of motion, including both top and bottom. These are the hardest reps and where it's most tempting to give up ownership.

Mass Mechanics Principle #2: The Principle of Respect

I learned this brilliant concept through RTS123.com. The phrase *"full range of motion"* is probably the most misused in bodybuilding. It's tossed around without considering that each of us has a unique body. We all have our own joint structure, length/tension relationships, and neural recruitment abilities. Not only that, but our body's abilities can vary from day to day and even set to set.

The principle of active and controllable range of motion means you only train through the range of motion that is available to you at each moment. Range of motion should never be determined by generic preset end points that you see someone else use. Just because someone in a video says to squat "ass to grass" does not mean you can or should. The body has built-in protective mechanisms to prevent injury. Some limitations are structural and set for life; others vary.

Growing up as a long-distance runner and triathlete, I was always taught that "tight muscles are bad" and that you need to stretch. A tight muscle is not necessarily a bad thing. The question is, why is it tight?

If a muscle is tight, it means something near it is weak, and you have to respect that (until you get it fixed). Many muscle imbalances can be worked through with Muscle Activation Techniques (MAT), which I'll discuss later on.

Before you begin any lift, determine what you can control based on your structure and current abilities. Don't lift any weight that's too heavy to control through your full range, or it's near certain you will increase wear and tear on the joints for zero net benefit. As a special bonus, to get access to a free video tutorial on how to access your active and controllable range of motion for all the major movement patterns, go to getlivinglarge.com/musclebonuses.

Key Concepts To Apply & Goals To Think About During Your Set

- *"Don't attempt to correct it. Just respect it."* Before you add any weight to an exercise, go through a full ROM practice rep to determine your "active and controllable" range of motion. Never disrespect these limits by adding weight and forcing yourself into a dangerous position that you can't control. Remember, if you can't control it, you can't challenge it.
- *"Listen to your body."* Your body uses this novel sensation called pain to motivate you to take an action—usually to protect body parts that your brain thinks are damaged, or about to be. If you feel any type of sensation or discomfort, it means your central nervous system thinks your body is under threat. If nothing is done to remove the "threat," your body turns up the "pain volume" until you must do something about it.

    Translated to the gym, a burning sensation in your muscles is the only pain that you should train through. If a certain grip/handle/stance/angle hurts your wrist, forearm, shoulder, hip, knee, ankle, etc., or causes any pain, then abandon it and find a position that allows you to lift pain free.

    People without the ability to feel pain (yes, they actually exist) don't live very long. If your body is speaking to you, listen![21]

Mass Mechanics Principle #3: The Principle of Disadvantages

Unlike other performance-based sports, the goal with weight training is to make every movement as hard as possible. You want to stay *inefficient*.

Building muscle is not about how much you lift or how many reps. It's about how well and how long you are able to keep the muscle under maximal tension.

Building muscle is not about how much you lift or how many reps. It's about how well and how long you are able to keep the muscle under maximal tension.

The easier the movement, the harder it is to build muscle because you're giving yourself an advantage. Training advantages do not build muscle; training disadvantages do.

If your goal is to lift heavier weights, use wrist straps and a weight belt. Give yourself that advantage. If you want to do 100 reps in 5 minutes, go ahead and swing it! Take the advantage of momentum! But to force your muscles to grow, you must make each rep, each set, and each workout as challenging as humanly possible.

The more disadvantages you present to the muscle, the more you force it to grow. Here are some key concepts to maximize tension and disadvantage within the muscle.

Key Concepts To Apply & Goals To Think About During Your Set:

- *"No pain, no gain."* Sometimes clichés are overused for a reason. When you maintain continuous tension through a muscle, weight training *hurts*. It's supposed to hurt. It's supposed to burn! Your *muscles* (not joints, tendons, or ligaments) are supposed to experience burning pain and skin-splitting pumps. You're supposed to feel like the lactic acid within the muscle can't escape. You're supposed to want to escape the pressure within the muscle. That's normal!

  Fight against mentally giving up too soon. Your body was made to withstand tremendous stress, so get comfortable with being uncomfortable. It's all about getting into The Hurt Box, an "insider" term my buddies and I used to reference "make or break moments" during grueling running workouts or the final leg of a race. The person who can go deep into The Hurt Box has a huge muscle-building edge. Yes, we must train smart, but training smart only works when you train hard!

- *"Lock it down."* Your body will always try to find a way to make the lift easier by shifting tension to surrounding muscle groups as you fatigue. This is known as cheating. We don't want any part of that. The next time you feel your form start to shift, think about "locking it down" to avoid losing tension in the targeted muscle.

- *"Avoid pausing at the top and bottom."* Unless the tempo prescribes otherwise, avoid making the set easier by pausing at the top or the bottom. The name of the game is continuous tension from the first rep to the last rep.

- *"Fully lengthen the muscle."* A muscle is fully lengthened when its antagonist (the opposite) is fully contracted. For instance, when you're doing an incline biceps curl, contract your triceps at the bottom of the range to ensure your biceps are fully lengthened before you initiate a contraction with the biceps. When doing lying leg curls, contract your quads at the bottom end of the range to ensure your hamstrings are fully lengthened before you engage them. Be prepared to use lighter weights.

- *"Fully shorten the muscle."* How do you know whether a muscle is fully shortened? It's fully contracted. In my experience most people are only contracting a muscle to 60 to 70 percent of their ability. They fail to understand that force is created internally, which is why concepts such as "squeeze it like it owes you money" are valuable. A great way to teach your brain to "fully shorten the muscle" is to pose and contract as hard as possible. Posing practice will translate into better contractile efficiency and shortening during your workouts and improve the "mind-muscle" connection. You shouldn't be able to hold an all-out contraction for much longer than 10 to 15 seconds. You'll know you're doing it right when your muscles cramp. Once you experience a maximal contraction without weights, your job is to replicate that same hard contraction, which will direct you to loads that you can control and own.

- *"Oppose the force."* Thanks to Isaac Newton, we know that for every action, there's an equal and opposite reaction. When you apply force in one direction, an opposing force will come along with it. You can use this principle to stabilize each exercise and prevent changes in form that would take tension off the targeted muscle. For example, shoving your shoulder blades into the bench before you do a chest press and keeping that pressure will force the back muscles to engage, which stabilizes the lift and helps keep tension in the chest muscles. During a T-bar row, if you lean back, you're using momentum to pull the weight, but if you shove your chest into the pad, you can lock your trunk into position, so that the target muscles get the maximum contraction. And when you train your lower body, for any closed-chain (your feet are touching something) leg movements, you should shove your feet into the ground or platform.

- *"Focus on the path of the joint, not the path of the dumbbell."* The shortest distance between two points is a straight line. The shortest distance to muscle growth is to use the fullest arc of the joint's range of motion that you can perform without pain. With each rep, this creates maximum muscle tissue tension at the extremes of the range. It also creates a greater training disadvantage and delivers a more purposeful workout. The goal here is to make the load adjust to your body, not to adjust your body to the load. We do this by identifying the invisible path the joint must travel, not the path of the dumbbell. If you just focus on moving the weight "up and down" and not taking the joint throughout its greatest arc, you'll miss out on "waking up" untrained muscle fibers at the extreme ends of the range, and you'll fail to develop your perceived "weak" body parts. The idea of "arcs" is a simple one to grasp when I describe it on video, which is a reason you should subscribe to my YouTube channel, youtube.com/vincedelmonte, where I show you how to maximize the arc for every exercise.

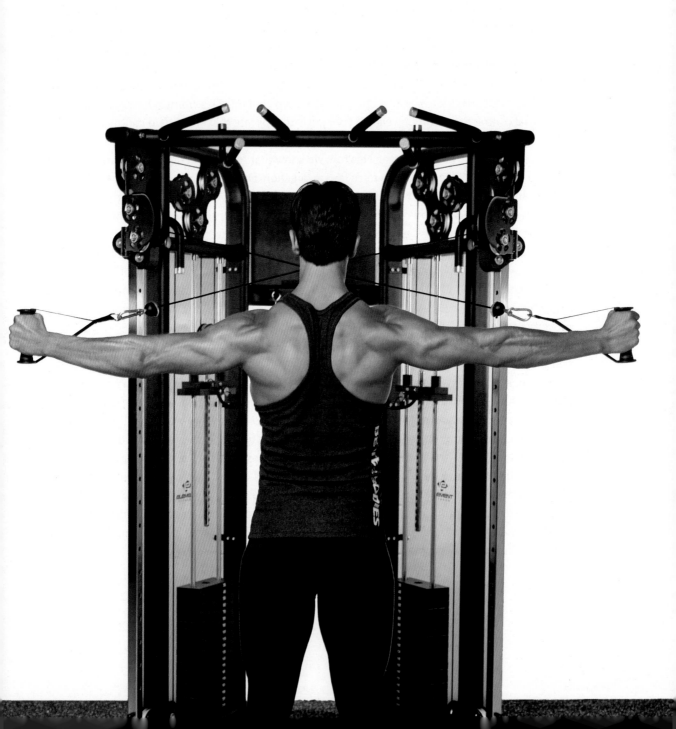

PART 6

The Ultimate 30-Week, Zero Guesswork Muscle-Building Program

What you are about to receive is 30 weeks of intelligently designed, step-by-step training programs that are 100 percent unique and that you won't find anywhere else. This is the program that delivers the training component to help you gain 30 pounds of pure muscle in the next 30 weeks.

I'm proud of this program. I had a lot of fun creating it. I believe it will be my greatest contribution to the skinny guy community.

Program Overview

In designing this program, I've taken the three mechanisms for muscle growth and integrated all of them into three 10-week phases to help you build your best body ever.

In Phase One, you will train your entire body three days a week and focus your entire workout for the day on Damage, Stress, or Tension, which means you will get three unique workouts this phase. In Phase Two, we move into a "Cube Rotation" where you will hit two major muscle groups hard and add a few "touch-up" sets for a few other muscle groups four times each week. Each workout is dedicated to either a Damage, Tension, or Stress Day, to provide you a total of twelve unique workouts in this phase. And finally, in Phase Three, you'll apply all three mechanisms while focusing on one major muscle group per workout and add a touch-up set on one other body part six times each workout, which means this phase gives you six more unique workouts.

Each phase contains nine weeks of hard training followed by one week of "de-loading," which is a purposeful reduction in training volume and intensity to improve performance, maximize muscle and strength gains, and prevent injury. To see a full overview of the entire 10 weeks, go to getlivinglarge.com/musclebonuses.

Here is some more information to help you follow the program.

Tempo

Tempo is a prescription for how long each phase of a repetition should last in seconds. There are four parts to every repetition. For example, a tempo may be written 4122.

Here are what the numbers mean, and which part of the repetition they correspond to:

- First number: Eccentric portion (when the load is going toward the floor)
- Second number: Pause in the stretched position between eccentric and concentric portions
- Third number: Concentric portion (when the load is moving away from the floor)
- Fourth number: Pause between repetitions

Note: *Any time there is an "X" in one of the four tempo slots, it means you are to perform that portion of the lift as explosively and powerfully as possible. For example, in order to perform a bench press on a 32X0 tempo, you would un-rack the barbell from the supports, take 3 seconds to lower it to your chest where you will pause for 2 seconds, then forcefully explode up as hard as possible with your arms extended, and go immediately into the next repetition.*

In another example, to perform chin-ups on a 4011 tempo, you take 4 seconds to lower your body from the bar, and with no pause at the bottom, pull your chest up to the bar in 1 second, then hold your chin over the bar for 1 second before lowering your body toward the floor on a 4 count.

Weight Selection

The sets prescribed are work sets, meaning you should be busting your butt.

You can do 1 or 2 warm-up sets prior to starting your first work set. The warm-up sets help you find an appropriate starting weight. On your Tension workout, if you need more than 1 to 2 warm-up sets, take them. There is no "right" or "wrong" number of warm-up sets. The goal is to prepare your muscles and brain for the first work set. Some days you may feel you need more and other days less.

The weight you select for your work sets is based on the reps, tempo, and rest period prescribed. If it says 6 to 8 reps, then that means 6 to 8 reps. If you can only do 5, it's too heavy. If you can do more than 8, it's too light (assuming you are following the prescribed tempo and rest periods). Don't overthink this.

The more you become familiar with your body, the easier it will be to select your weights. Be sure to record what you do, so you have a range to gun for at the next workout.

Rest Periods

The rest periods indicate how much you should rest between each set and between each exercise. A 60-second rest means a 60-second rest. It doesn't mean you start getting ready for the next set after 60 seconds; it means you start the next set 60 seconds after you completed the final rep of your previous set. This requires a stopwatch.

Sometimes, I indicate rest periods with ranges that give you the flexibility to customize the intensity.

Exercise Order

Do all the sets of one exercise in a row (with rest periods between each set) before moving on to the next exercise.

A1:A2 represents a super set, which means you will do both exercises back-to-back before resting and repeating.

A1:A2:A3 represents a giant set, which means you will do all three exercises back-to-back before resting and repeating.

I realize I just gave you a lot to absorb, so you might want to read through this a few times to get familiar. It will all make more sense once you get in the gym.

Trust the program. Follow it. Everything here has a reason to be and has been well thought out. I reassure you that there are no typos in this program. Pick a start date, ideally this coming Monday. Track your workouts.

Enjoy the journey. I can't wait to see your results!

Phase One

Objective

The goal of this phase is to expose your body to the three mechanisms that contribute to hypertrophy: muscular damage, mechanical tension, and metabolic stress. In this phase, you will train three times per week doing full body workouts. Each session is focused on one of the three mechanisms.

For the mechanical tension workouts, focus on lifting heavy weights with full recovery. Do not shorten the rest periods even if you feel inclined to do so. The more weight you can load while maintaining proper technique, the more tension you will create. Aim to increase your loads each week as you make your way through this first phase. Big barbell lifts are key in this workout.

For the metabolic stress workouts, you will shoot for high reps and take short rest periods. Expect to feel a big burn in this phase! The more burn you feel, the more metabolites are present in your bloodstream. These metabolites are powerful signalers for muscle growth, so learn to embrace the burn! We will mainly use machines and isolation moves for this phase, so that you don't have to worry too much about balance, and you can fully fatigue the targeted muscles.

Finally, in the damage workouts, you will lift heavy weights with a slow eccentric (lowering) component. Eccentric stress creates a lot of muscle damage, which is critical for maximizing hypertrophy. Many of these exercises are done in the stretched position, making them even more effective at creating muscle damage.

Training Split

The recommended split for this phase is:

- Monday – Workout One
- Tuesday – Off
- Wednesday – Workout Two
- Thursday – Off
- Friday – Workout Three
- Saturday – Off
- Sunday – Off

Intensity Technique

*Drop Sets: *On your full body stress days, pay attention to the last set of each exercise, where you will be asked to reduce the weight and do more reps. This technique progresses every 4 weeks and is outlined below.*

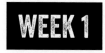

Workout One - Full Body Tension

ORDER	EXERCISE	SETS	REPS	TEMPO	REST
A	Barbell Back Squat	3	6-8	30X0	2-3 min
B	Mid-Grip Barbell Shoulder Press in Front	3	6-8	30X0	2-3 min
C	Clean Grip Deadlift	3	6-8	31X0	2-3 min
D	Barbell Bench Press	3	6-8	30X0	2-3 min
E	Narrow Grip Neutral Chin-Up	3	6-8	30X1	2-3 min
F	Dips (torso upright)	3	6-8	30X0	2-3 min
G	Standing Barbell Curl	3	6-8	30X0	2-3 min

Workout Two - Full Body Stress

ORDER	EXERCISE	SETS	REPS	TEMPO	REST
A	Leg Press	3	20*	2010	60 sec
B	Neutral Grip Seated Cable Row	3	20*	2011	60 sec
C	Push-Up	3	20*	2011	60 sec
D	Low Pulley Pull Through	3	20*	2010	60 sec
E	Low Pulley Upright Row with Rope	3	20*	2011	60 sec
F	Triceps Pressdown with Rope	3	20*	2011	60 sec
G	Standing Dumbbell (DB) Hammer Curl	3	20*	2010	60 sec

*Drop Set: *On your last set of each exercise, do your hard 20 reps, then immediately decrease the weight 10 to 15 percent and do another 20 reps to finish that exercise. For the push-ups, drop to your knees for the drop set.*

Workout Three - Full Body Damage

ORDER	EXERCISE	SETS	REPS	TEMPO	REST
A	Barbell Front Squat	3	8-10	60X0	90 sec
B	Incline DB Bench Press	3	8-10	60X0	90 sec
C	Lying Leg Curl	3	8-10	60X0	90 sec
D	Wide Grip Pronated Pull-Up	3	8-10	60X0	90 sec
E	Kneeling Low Pulley French Press with Rope (overhead triceps extension)	3	8-10	60X0	90 sec
F	Incline DB Curl	3	8-10	60X0	90 sec
G	Seated 2-Arm DB Lateral Raise	3	8-10	60X0	90 sec

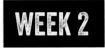

Workout One – Full Body Tension

ORDER	EXERCISE	SETS	REPS	TEMPO	REST
A	Barbell Back Squat	3	6-8	30X0	2-3 min
B	Mid-Grip Barbell Shoulder Press in Front	3	6-8	30X0	2-3 min
C	Clean Grip Deadlift	3	6-8	31X0	2-3 min
D	Barbell Bench Press	3	6-8	30X0	2-3 min
E	Narrow Grip Neutral Chin-Up	3	6-8	30X1	2-3 min
F	Dips (torso upright)	3	6-8	30X0	2-3 min
G	Standing Barbell Curl	3	6-8	30X0	2-3 min

Workout Two – Full Body Stress

ORDER	EXERCISE	SETS	REPS	TEMPO	REST
A	Leg Press	3	20*	2010	60 sec
B	Neutral Grip Seated Cable Row	3	20*	2011	60 sec
C	Push-Up	3	20*	2011	60 sec
D	Low Pulley Pull Through	3	20*	2010	60 sec
E	Low Pulley Upright Row with Rope	3	20*	2011	60 sec
F	Triceps Pressdown with Rope	3	20*	2011	60 sec
G	Standing DB Hammer Curl	3	20*	2010	60 sec

*Drop Set: *On your last set of each exercise, do your hard 20 reps, then immediately decrease the weight 10 to 15 percent and do another 20 reps to finish that exercise. For the push-ups, drop to your knees for the drop set.*

Workout Three – Full Body Damage

ORDER	EXERCISE	SETS	REPS	TEMPO	REST
A	Barbell Front Squat	3	8-10	60X0	90 sec
B	Incline DB Bench Press	3	8-10	60X0	90 sec
C	Lying Leg Curl	3	8-10	60X0	90 sec
D	Wide Grip Pronated Pull-Up	3	8-10	60X0	90 sec
E	Kneeling Low Pulley French Press with Rope (overhead triceps extension)	3	8-10	60X0	90 sec
F	Incline DB Curl	3	8-10	60X0	90 sec
G	Seated 2-Arm DB Lateral Raise	3	8-10	60X0	90 sec

WEEK 3

Workout One - Full Body Tension

ORDER	EXERCISE	SETS	REPS	TEMPO	REST
A	Barbell Back Squat	3	6-8	30X0	2-3 min
B	Mid-Grip Barbell Shoulder Press in Front	3	6-8	30X0	2-3 min
C	Clean Grip Deadlift	3	6-8	31X0	2-3 min
D	Barbell Bench Press	3	6-8	30X0	2-3 min
E	Narrow Grip Neutral Chin-Up	3	6-8	30X1	2-3 min
F	Dips (torso upright)	3	6-8	30X0	2-3 min
G	Standing Barbell Curl	3	6-8	30X0	2-3 min

Workout Two - Full Body Stress

ORDER	EXERCISE	SETS	REPS	TEMPO	REST
A	Leg Press	3	20*	2010	60 sec
B	Neutral Grip Seated Cable Row	3	20*	2011	60 sec
C	Push-Up	3	20*	2011	60 sec
D	Low Pulley Pull Through	3	20*	2010	60 sec
E	Low Pulley Upright Row with Rope	3	20*	2011	60 sec
F	Triceps Pressdown with Rope	3	20*	2011	60 sec
G	Standing DB Hammer Curl	3	20*	2010	60 sec

*Drop Set: *On your last set of each exercise, do your hard 20 reps, then immediately decrease the weight 10 to 15 percent and do another 20 reps to finish that exercise. For the push-ups, drop to your knees for the drop set.*

Workout Three - Full Body Damage

ORDER	EXERCISE	SETS	REPS	TEMPO	REST
A	Barbell Front Squat	3	8-10	60X0	90 sec
B	Incline DB Bench Press	3	8-10	60X0	90 sec
C	Lying Leg Curl	3	8-10	60X0	90 sec
D	Wide Grip Pronated Pull-Up	3	8-10	60X0	90 sec
E	Kneeling Low Pulley French Press with Rope (overhead triceps extension)	3	8-10	60X0	90 sec
F	Incline DB Curl	3	8-10	60X0	90 sec
G	Seated 2-Arm DB Lateral Raise	3	8-10	60X0	90 sec

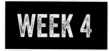

Workout One - Full Body Tension

ORDER	EXERCISE	SETS	REPS	TEMPO	REST
A	Barbell Back Squat	3	5	30X0	2-3 min
B	Mid-Grip Barbell Shoulder Press in Front	3	5	30X0	2-3 min
C	Clean Grip Deadlift	3	5	31X0	2-3 min
D	Barbell Bench Press	3	5	30X0	2-3 min
E	Narrow Grip Neutral Chin-Up	3	5	30X1	2-3 min
F	Dips (torso upright)	3	5	30X0	2-3 min
G	Standing Barbell Curl	3	5	30X0	2-3 min

Workout Two - Full Body Stress

ORDER	EXERCISE	SETS	REPS	TEMPO	REST
A	Leg Press	3	15*	2010	60 sec
B	Neutral Grip Seated Cable Row	3	15*	2011	60 sec
C	Push-Up	3	15*	2011	60 sec
D	Low Pulley Pull Through	3	15*	2010	60 sec
E	Low Pulley Upright Row with Rope	3	15*	2011	60 sec
F	Triceps Pressdown with Rope	3	15*	2011	60 sec
G	Standing DB Hammer Curl	3	15*	2010	60 sec

Drop Set: *On your last set of each exercise, do your hard 15 reps, then immediately decrease the weight 8 to 12 percent and do another 15, then decrease the weight another 10 to 15 percent and do 15 reps to finish that exercise, for 45 reps total in your final set. For the push-ups, drop to your knees for the first drop set and widen your hands for the second drop set.*

Workout Three - Full Body Damage

ORDER	EXERCISE	SETS	REPS	TEMPO	REST
A	Barbell Front Squat	3	7-9	70X0	90 sec
B	Incline DB Bench Press	3	7-9	70X0	90 sec
C	Lying Leg Curl	3	7-9	70X0	90 sec
D	Wide Grip Pronated Pull-Up	3	7-9	70X0	90 sec
E	Kneeling Low Pulley French Press with Rope (overhead triceps extension)	3	7-9	70X0	90 sec
F	Incline DB Curl	3	7-9	70X0	90 sec
G	Seated 2-Arm DB Lateral Raise	3	7-9	70X0	90 sec

WEEK 5

Workout One - Full Body Tension

ORDER	EXERCISE	SETS	REPS	TEMPO	REST
A	Barbell Back Squat	3	5	30X0	2-3 min
B	Mid-Grip Barbell Shoulder Press in Front	3	5	30X0	2-3 min
C	Clean Grip Deadlift	3	5	31X0	2-3 min
D	Barbell Bench Press	3	5	30X0	2-3 min
E	Narrow Grip Neutral Chin-Up	3	5	30X1	2-3 min
F	Dips (torso upright)	3	5	30X0	2-3 min
G	Standing Barbell Curl	3	5	30X0	2-3 min

Workout Two - Full Body Stress

ORDER	EXERCISE	SETS	REPS	TEMPO	REST
A	Leg Press	3	15*	2010	60 sec
B	Neutral Grip Seated Cable Row	3	15*	2011	60 sec
C	Push-Up	3	15*	2011	60 sec
D	Low Pulley Pull Through	3	15*	2010	60 sec
E	Low Pulley Upright Row with Rope	3	15*	2011	60 sec
F	Triceps Pressdown with Rope	3	15*	2011	60 sec
G	Standing DB Hammer Curl	3	15*	2010	60 sec

*__*Drop Set:__ On your last set of each exercise, do your hard 15 reps, then immediately decrease the weight 8 to 12 percent and do another 15, then decrease the weight another 10 to 15 percent and do 15 reps to finish that exercise, for 45 reps total in your final set. For the push-ups, drop to your knees for the first drop set and widen your hands for the second drop set.*

Workout Three - Full Body Damage

ORDER	EXERCISE	SETS	REPS	TEMPO	REST
A	Barbell Front Squat	3	7-9	70X0	90 sec
B	Incline DB Bench Press	3	7-9	70X0	90 sec
C	Lying Leg Curl	3	7-9	70X0	90 sec
D	Wide Grip Pronated Pull-Up	3	7-9	70X0	90 sec
E	Kneeling Low Pulley French Press with Rope (overhead triceps extension)	3	7-9	70X0	90 sec
F	Incline DB Curl	3	7-9	70X0	90 sec
G	Seated 2-Arm DB Lateral Raise	3	7-9	70X0	90 sec

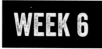

Workout One - Full Body Tension

ORDER	EXERCISE	SETS	REPS	TEMPO	REST
A	Barbell Back Squat	3	5	30X0	2-3 min
B	Mid-Grip Barbell Shoulder Press in Front	3	5	30X0	2-3 min
C	Clean Grip Deadlift	3	5	31X0	2-3 min
D	Barbell Bench Press	3	5	30X0	2-3 min
E	Narrow Grip Neutral Chin-Up	3	5	30X1	2-3 min
F	Dips (torso upright)	3	5	30X0	2-3 min
G	Standing Barbell Curl	3	5	30X0	2-3 min

Workout Two - Full Body Stress

ORDER	EXERCISE	SETS	REPS	TEMPO	REST
A	Leg Press	3	15*	2010	60 sec
B	Neutral Grip Seated Cable Row	3	15*	2011	60 sec
C	Push-Up	3	15*	2011	60 sec
D	Low Pulley Pull Through	3	15*	2010	60 sec
E	Low Pulley Upright Row with Rope	3	15*	2011	60 sec
F	Triceps Pressdown with Rope	3	15*	2011	60 sec
G	Standing DB Hammer Curl	3	15*	2010	60 sec

Drop Set: On your last set of each exercise, do your hard 15 reps, then immediately decrease the weight 8 to 12 percent and do another 15, then decrease the weight another 10 to 15 percent and do 15 reps to finish that exercise, for 45 reps total in your final set. For the push-ups, drop to your knees for the first drop set and widen your hands for the second drop set.

Workout Three - Full Body Damage

ORDER	EXERCISE	SETS	REPS	TEMPO	REST
A	Barbell Front Squat	3	7-9	70X0	90 sec
B	Incline DB Bench Press	3	7-9	70X0	90 sec
C	Lying Leg Curl	3	7-9	70X0	90 sec
D	Wide Grip Pronated Pull-Up	3	7-9	70X0	90 sec
E	Kneeling Low Pulley French Press with Rope (overhead triceps extension)	3	7-9	70X0	90 sec
F	Incline DB Curl	3	7-9	70X0	90 sec
G	Seated 2-Arm DB Lateral Raise	3	7-9	70X0	90 sec

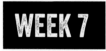

Workout One - Full Body Tension

ORDER	EXERCISE	SETS	REPS	TEMPO	REST
A	Barbell Back Squat	4	4	30X0	2-3 min
B	Mid-Grip Barbell Shoulder Press in Front	4	4	30X0	2-3 min
C	Clean Grip Deadlift	4	4	31X0	2-3 min
D	Barbell Bench Press	4	4	30X0	2-3 min
E	Narrow Grip Neutral Chin-Up	4	4	30X1	2-3 min
F	Dips (torso upright)	4	4	30X0	2-3 min
G	Standing Barbell Curl	4	4	30X0	2-3 min

Workout Two - Full Body Stress

ORDER	EXERCISE	SETS	REPS	TEMPO	REST
A	Leg Press	3	10*	2010	60 sec
B	Neutral Grip Seated Cable Row	3	10*	2011	60 sec
C	Push-Up	3	10*	2011	60 sec
D	Low Pulley Pull Through	3	10*	2010	60 sec
E	Low Pulley Upright Row with Rope	3	10*	2011	60 sec
F	Triceps Pressdown with Rope	3	10*	2011	60 sec
G	Standing DB Hammer Curl	3	10*	2010	60 sec

*Drop Set: *On your last set of each exercise, do your hard 10 reps, then immediately decrease the weight 5 to 7 percent and do another 10 reps, then decrease the weight another 8 to 10 percent and do another 10 reps, and then drop another 10 percent of the weight and do 10 reps to finish that exercise, for 40 reps total in your final set. For the push-ups, drop to your knees for the first drop set and widen your hands for the second and third drop set.*

Workout Three - Full Body Damage

ORDER	EXERCISE	SETS	REPS	TEMPO	REST
A	Barbell Front Squat	3	6-8	80X0	90 sec
B	Incline DB Bench Press	3	6-8	80X0	90 sec
C	Lying Leg Curl	3	6-8	80X0	90 sec
D	Wide Grip Pronated Pull-Up	3	6-8	80X0	90 sec
E	Kneeling Low Pulley French Press with Rope (overhead triceps extension)	3	6-8	80X0	90 sec
F	Incline DB Curl	3	6-8	80X0	90 sec
G	Seated 2-Arm DB Lateral Raise	3	6-8	80X0	90 sec

WEEK 8

Workout One – Full Body Tension

ORDER	EXERCISE	SETS	REPS	TEMPO	REST
A	Barbell Back Squat	4	4	30X0	2–3 min
B	Mid-Grip Barbell Shoulder Press in Front	4	4	30X0	2–3 min
C	Clean Grip Deadlift	4	4	31X0	2–3 min
D	Barbell Bench Press	4	4	30X0	2–3 min
E	Narrow Grip Neutral Chin-Up	4	4	30X1	2–3 min
F	Dips (torso upright)	4	4	30X0	2–3 min
G	Standing Barbell Curl	4	4	30X0	2–3 min

Workout Two – Full Body Stress

ORDER	EXERCISE	SETS	REPS	TEMPO	REST
A	Leg Press	3	10*	2010	60 sec
B	Neutral Grip Seated Cable Row	3	10*	2011	60 sec
C	Push-Up	3	10*	2011	60 sec
D	Low Pulley Pull Through	3	10*	2010	60 sec
E	Low Pulley Upright Row with Rope	3	10*	2011	60 sec
F	Triceps Pressdown with Rope	3	10*	2011	60 sec
G	Standing DB Hammer Curl	3	10*	2010	60 sec

Drop Set: On your last set of each exercise, do your hard 10 reps, then immediately decrease the weight 5 to 7 percent and do another 10 reps, then decrease the weight another 8 to 10 percent and do another 10 reps, and then drop another 10 percent of the weight and do 10 reps to finish that exercise, for 40 reps total in your final set.
For the push-ups, drop to your knees for the first drop set and widen your hands for the second and third drop set.

Workout Three – Full Body Damage

ORDER	EXERCISE	SETS	REPS	TEMPO	REST
A	Barbell Front Squat	3	6–8	80X0	90 sec
B	Incline DB Bench Press	3	6–8	80X0	90 sec
C	Lying Leg Curl	3	6–8	80X0	90 sec
D	Wide Grip Pronated Pull-Up	3	6–8	80X0	90 sec
E	Kneeling Low Pulley French Press with Rope (overhead triceps extension)	3	6–8	80X0	90 sec
F	Incline DB Curl	3	6–8	80X0	90 sec
G	Seated 2-Arm DB Lateral Raise	3	6–8	80X0	90 sec

Workout One – Full Body Tension

ORDER	EXERCISE	SETS	REPS	TEMPO	REST
A	Barbell Back Squat	4	4	30X0	2-3 min
B	Mid-Grip Barbell Shoulder Press in Front	4	4	30X0	2-3 min
C	Clean Grip Deadlift	4	4	31X0	2-3 min
D	Barbell Bench Press	4	4	30X0	2-3 min
E	Narrow Grip Neutral Chin-Up	4	4	30X1	2-3 min
F	Dips (torso upright)	4	4	30X0	2-3 min
G	Standing Barbell Curl	4	4	30X0	2-3 min

Workout Two – Full Body Stress

ORDER	EXERCISE	SETS	REPS	TEMPO	REST
A	Leg Press	3	10*	2010	60 sec
B	Neutral Grip Seated Cable Row	3	10*	2011	60 sec
C	Push-Up	3	10*	2011	60 sec
D	Low Pulley Pull Through	3	10*	2010	60 sec
E	Low Pulley Upright Row with Rope	3	10*	2011	60 sec
F	Triceps Pressdown with Rope	3	10*	2011	60 sec
G	Standing DB Hammer Curl	3	10*	2010	60 sec

***Drop Set:** On your last set of each exercise, do your hard 10 reps, then immediately decrease the weight 5 to 7 percent and do another 10 reps, then decrease the weight another 8 to 10 percent and do another 10 reps, and then drop another 10 percent of the weight and do 10 reps to finish that exercise, for 40 reps total in your final set. For the push-ups, drop to your knees for the first drop set and widen your hands for the second and third drop set.*

Workout Three – Full Body Damage

ORDER	EXERCISE	SETS	REPS	TEMPO	REST
A	Barbell Front Squat	3	6-8	80X0	90 sec
B	Incline DB Bench Press	3	6-8	80X0	90 sec
C	Lying Leg Curl	3	6-8	80X0	90 sec
D	Wide Grip Pronated Pull-Up	3	6-8	80X0	90 sec
E	Kneeling Low Pulley French Press with Rope (overhead triceps extension)	3	6-8	80X0	90 sec
F	Incline DB Curl	3	6-8	80X0	90 sec
G	Seated 2-Arm DB Lateral Raise	3	6-8	80X0	90 sec

WEEK 10 – UNLOADING WEEK

Workout One - Full Body Tension

ORDER	EXERCISE	SETS	REPS	TEMPO	REST
A	Barbell Back Squat	1	4	30X0	2–3 min
B	Mid-Grip Barbell Shoulder Press in Front	1	4	30X0	2–3 min
C	Clean Grip Deadlift	1	4	31X0	2–3 min
D	Barbell Bench Press	1	4	30X0	2–3 min
E	Narrow Grip Neutral Chin-Up	1	4	30X1	2–3 min
F	Dips (torso upright)	1	4	30X0	2–3 min
G	Standing Barbell Curl	1	4	30X0	2–3 min

Workout Two - Full Body Stress

ORDER	EXERCISE	SETS	REPS	TEMPO	REST
A	Leg Press	1	10	2010	60 sec
B	Neutral Grip Seated Cable Row	1	10	2011	60 sec
C	Push-Up	1	10	2011	60 sec
D	Low Pulley Pull Through	1	10	2010	60 sec
E	Low Pulley Upright Row with Rope	1	10	2011	60 sec
F	Triceps Pressdown with Rope	1	10	2011	60 sec
G	Standing DB Hammer Curl	1	10	2010	60 sec

Note: *No drop sets this week*

Workout Three - Full Body Damage

ORDER	EXERCISE	SETS	REPS	TEMPO	REST
A	Barbell Front Squat	1	6–8	80X0	90 sec
B	Incline DB Bench Press	1	6–8	80X0	90 sec
C	Lying Leg Curl	1	6–8	80X0	90 sec
D	Wide Grip Pronated Pull-Up	1	6–8	80X0	90 sec
E	Kneeling Low Pulley French Press with Rope (overhead triceps extension)	1	6–8	80X0	90 sec
F	Incline DB Curl	1	6–8	80X0	90 sec
G	Seated 2-Arm DB Lateral Raise	1	6–8	80X0	90 sec

Phase Two

Objective

In this phase, we will continue to trigger you to the three mechanisms of muscle growth, but in a different way. This time, you will rotate through workouts that focus on each mechanism.

You will train four times per week in this phase, with a main workout focused on each body part and a few "touch-up" sets for a few other muscle groups. These touch-up sets allow you to spread the volume over two workouts per week and give you a twice-per-week stimulus per body part, which is the perfect frequency for maximal hypertrophy.

Training Split

- Monday: Chest and Back (Shoulders and Arms Touch-Up)
- Tuesday: Quads and Calves (Hamstrings and Abs Touch-Up)
- Wednesday: Off
- Thursday: Shoulders and Arms (Chest and Back Touch-Up)
- Friday: Hamstrings and Abs (Quads and Calves Touch-Up)
- Saturday: Off
- Sunday: Off

Maintain the split above for the entire phase, but rotate which workouts you do.

There are three different workouts for each body part to cycle through for the main body part of each session. You'll do each workout three times in this phase, and you should strive to outperform your previous week's workout by adding load (with good technique, of course) each time you repeat the workout. The best way to visualize this is to write the split on your calendar. Then, go through, starting with the first workout and going in order, and write "Tension," "Damage," "Stress," "Tension," "Damage," "Stress," etc., from workout to workout to the end of the cycle.

The cycle will repeat itself in weeks 4 to 6 and again in weeks 7 to 9. In week 10, you will do a very simple unloading week to get ready for phase three. You can find your unloading workouts (which you will do for each body part that week) at the end of this phase's workouts.

Here's a full cube rotation schedule of the first three weeks so that you can see what I mean.

WEEK 1

- Monday: Chest and Back – Tension Workout
- Tuesday: Quads and Calves – Damage Workout
- Wednesday: Off
- Thursday: Shoulders and Arms – Stress Workout

- Friday: Hamstrings and Abs – Tension Workout
- Saturday: Off
- Sunday: Off

WEEK 2

- Monday: Chest and Back – Damage Workout
- Tuesday: Quads and Calves – Stress Workout
- Wednesday: Off
- Thursday: Shoulders and Arms – Tension Workout
- Friday: Hamstrings and Abs – Damage Workout
- Saturday: Off
- Sunday: Off

WEEK 3

- Monday: Chest and Back – Stress Workout
- Tuesday: Quads and Calves – Tension Workout
- Wednesday: Off
- Thursday: Shoulders and Arms – Damage Workout
- Friday: Hamstrings and Abs – Stress Workout
- Saturday: Off
- Sunday: Off

WEEKS 4, 5, AND 6   and   WEEKS 7, 8, AND 9

Repeat weeks 1 through 3 in order.

WEEK 10

Repeat unloading.

Intensity Technique: *For the 2 up / 1 down technique, lift the weight with 2 arms, and then lower under control using only 1 limb with the proper eccentric tempo. Do 1 complete set with 1 limb before switching sides. This will make you very sore!*

CHEST AND BACK WORKOUTS (SHOULDERS AND ARMS TOUCH-UP)

Chest and Back Tension Workout (Shoulders and Arms Touch-Up)

ORDER	EXERCISE	SETS	REPS	TEMPO	REST
A1	Incline Barbell Bench Press	10	5	30X0	90 sec
A2	Wide Grip Pronated Pull-Up	10	5	30X0	90 sec
B1	Lean-Away DB Lateral Raise	2	8-10	3011	10 sec
B2	Low Pulley Rope Curl	2	8-10	30X0	10 sec
B3	EZ Bar Triceps Extension	2	8-10	30X1	60 sec

Chest and Back Damage Workout (Shoulders and Arms Touch-Up)

ORDER	EXERCISE	SETS	REPS	TEMPO	REST
A1	Machine Chest Press (2 up / 1 down technique*)	8	6 ea	80X0	90 sec
A2	Machine Row (2 up / 1 down technique*)	8	6 ea	80X0	90 sec
B1	Lean-Away DB Lateral Raise	2	8-10	3011	10 sec
B2	Low Pulley Rope Curl	2	8-10	30X0	10 sec
B3	EZ Bar Triceps Extension	2	8-10	30X1	60 sec

For the 2 up / 1 down technique, lift the weight with two arms, and then lower under control using only one limb with the proper eccentric tempo. Do 1 complete set with 1 limb before switching sides. This will make you very sore!

Chest and Back Stress Workout (Shoulders and Arms Touch-Up)

ORDER	EXERCISE	SETS	REPS	TEMPO	REST
A1	Incline Press Machine	3	12-15	3011	10 sec
A2	DB Chest Fly	3	12-15	2210	10 sec
A3	Low Pulley Dual Cable Incline Fly	3	12-15	2011	10 sec
A4	Pec Deck Chest Fly	3	12-15	2011	90 sec
B1	Supinated Grip Seated Cable Row	3	12-15	3010	10 sec
B2	Mid-Grip Supinated Lat Pulldown	3	12-15	3011	10 sec
B3	Prone Incline 2-Arm DB Row	3	12-15	2011	10 sec
B4	DB Pullover on Flat Bench	3	12-15	3030	90 sec
C1	Lean-Away DB Lateral Raise	2	8-10	3011	10 sec
C2	Low Pulley Rope Curl	2	8-10	30X0	10 sec
C3	EZ Bar Triceps Extension	2	8-10	30X1	60 sec

QUADS AND CALVES WORKOUTS (HAMSTRINGS AND ABS TOUCH-UP)

Quads and Calves Tension Workout (Hamstrings and Abs Touch-Up)

ORDER	EXERCISE	SETS	REPS	TEMPO	REST
A1	Heels Elevated Barbell Back Squat	10	5	30X0	60 sec
A2	Standing Calf Raise Machine	10	10	2112	3 min
B1	Med-Ball or Weight Plate V-Up	2	8-10	3011	10 sec
B2	Lying Leg Curl	2	8-10	30X1	60 sec

Quads and Calves Damage Workout (Hamstrings and Abs Touch-Up)

ORDER	EXERCISE	SETS	REPS	TEMPO	REST
A1	Leg Extension (2 up / 1 down technique*)	8	6 ea	80X0	90 sec
A2	Standing Calf Raise Machine (2 up / 1 down technique*)	8	6 ea	80X0	90 sec
B1	Med-Ball or Weight Plate V-Up	2	8-10	3011	10 sec
B2	Lying Leg Curl	2	8-10	30X1	60 sec

For the 2 up / 1 down technique, lift the weight with two arms, and then lower under control using only one limb with the proper eccentric tempo. Do 1 complete set with 1 limb before switching sides. This will make you very sore!

Quads and Calves Stress Workout (Hamstrings and Abs Touch-Up)

ORDER	EXERCISE	SETS	REPS	TEMPO	REST
A1	Hack Squat Machine	3	12-15	3011	10 sec
A2	Alternating Barbell Lunge	3	12-15	2210	10 sec
A3	Heels Elevated DB Squat	3	12-15	2011	10 sec
A4	DB Bulgarian Split Squat (rear foot elevated)	3	12-15	2011	90 sec
B1	Seated Calf Raise (toes neutral)	3	12-15	3010	10 sec
B2	Standing Calf Raise Machine	3	12-15	3011	10 sec
B3	Toe Press (calf raise on leg press machine)	3	12-15	2011	10 sec
B4	Body weight 1-Leg Calf Raise	3	12-15	3030	90 sec
C1	Med-Ball or Weight Plate V-Up	2	8-10	3011	10 sec
C2	Lying Leg Curl	2	8-10	30X1	60 sec

SHOULDERS AND ARMS WORKOUTS (CHEST AND BACK TOUCH-UP)

Shoulders and Arms Tension Workout (Chest and Back Touch-Up)

ORDER	EXERCISE	SETS	REPS	TEMPO	REST
A	Seated DB Shoulder Press	10	5	30X0	100 sec
B1	Close Grip Barbell Bench Press (shoulder width)	10	5	30X0	75 sec
B2	Mid-Grip Straight Bar Scott Curl	10	5	30X0	75 sec
C1	Pec Deck Chest Fly	2	8-10	2012	10 sec
C2	DB Pullover on Flat Bench	2	8-10	3020	60 sec

Shoulders and Arms Damage Workout (Chest and Back Touch-Up)

ORDER	EXERCISE	SETS	REPS	TEMPO	REST
A1	Eccentric Emphasis "L" Lateral Raise	8	6	80X0	60 sec
A2	Machine Curl (2 up / 1 down technique*)	8	6 ea	80X0	60 sec
A3	Triceps Extension Machine (2 up / 1 down technique*)	8	6 ea	80X0	60 sec
B1	Pec Deck Chest Fly	2	8-10	2012	10 sec
B2	DB Pullover on Flat Bench	2	8-10	3020	60 sec

For the 2 up / 1 down technique, lift the weight with two arms, and then lower under control using only one limb with the proper eccentric tempo. Do 1 complete set with 1 limb before switching sides. This will make you very sore!

Shoulders and Arms Stress Workout (Chest and Back Touch-Up)

ORDER	EXERCISE	SETS	REPS	TEMPO	REST
A1	Seated EZ Bar French Press (overhead triceps extension)	3	12-15	31X0	10 sec
A2	Triceps Pressdown with Rope	3	12-15	3011	10 sec
A3	EZ Bar Triceps Extension	3	12-15	2011	10 sec
A4	Shoulder Width Push-Up	3	Max reps	20X0	60 sec
B1	Mid-Grip Straight Bar Scott Curl	3	12-15	3010	10 sec
B2	Standing Barbell Drag Curl	3	12-15	3011	10 sec
B3	Incline DB Hammer Curl	3	12-15	2011	10 sec
B4	Low Pulley Rope Curl	3	12-15	N/A	60 sec
C1	Seated DB Shoulder Press	3	12-15	2011	10 sec
C2	Snatch Grip Upright Row	3	12-15	2011	10 sec

CONTINUED

ORDER	EXERCISE	SETS	REPS	TEMPO	REST
	[CONTINUED]				
C3	Prone Steep Incline DB Lateral Raise	3	12-15	2011	10 sec
C4	Rear Delt on Pec Fly Machine	3	12-15	2011	60 sec
D1	Pec Deck Chest Fly	2	8-10	2012	10 sec
D2	DB Pullover on Flat Bench	2	8-10	3020	60 sec

HAMSTRINGS AND ABS WORKOUTS (QUADS AND CALVES TOUCH-UP)

Hamstrings and Abs Tension Workout (Quads and Calves Touch-Up)

ORDER	EXERCISE	SETS	REPS	TEMPO	REST
A1	Snatch Grip Deadlift	10	5	30X0	60 sec
A2	Hanging Garhammer Raise (90 degrees and up)	10	15-20	2012	3 min
B1	Standing Calf Raise Machine	2	8-10	1011	10 sec
B2	DB Bulgarian Split Squat (rear foot elevated)	2	8-10 ea	30X1	60 sec

Hamstrings and Abs Damage Workout (Quads and Calves Touch-Up)

ORDER	EXERCISE	SETS	REPS	TEMPO	REST
A1	Lying Leg Curl (2 up / 1 down technique*)	8	6 ea	80X0	90 sec
A2	Hanging Garhammer Raise (90 degrees and up)	8	6	80X0	90 sec
B1	Standing Calf Raise Machine	2	8-10	1011	10 sec
B2	DB Bulgarian Split Squat (rear foot elevated)	2	8-10 ea	30X1	60 sec

For the 2 up / 1 down technique, lift the weight with two arms, and then lower under control using only one limb with the proper eccentric tempo. Do 1 complete set with 1 limb before switching sides. This will make you very sore!

Hamstrings and Abs Stress Workout (Quads and Calves Touch-Up)

ORDER	EXERCISE	SETS	REPS	TEMPO	REST
A1	Barbell RDL	3	12-15	30X0	10 sec
A2	Swiss Ball Hip Bridge / Leg Curl Combo	3	12-15	2020	10 sec
A3	Horizontal Back Extension	3	12-15	2011	10 sec
A4	Lying Leg Curl	3	12-15	2011	90 sec
B1	Hanging Garhammer Raise (90 degrees and up)	3	12-15	3010	10 sec
B2	Med-Ball or Weight Plate V-Up	3	12-15	3011	10 sec

ORDER	EXERCISE	SETS	REPS	TEMPO	REST
B3	Front Plank	3	Max time	2011	10 sec
B4	Side Plank	3	Max time ea	N/A	90 sec
C1	Standing Calf Raise Machine	2	8-10	1011	10 sec
C2	DB Bulgarian Split Squat (rear foot elevated)	2	8-10 ea	30X1	60 sec

WEEK 10 UNLOADING WEEK WORKOUTS

Chest and Back Unloading Workout (Shoulders and Arms Touch-Up)

ORDER	EXERCISE	SETS	REPS	TEMPO	REST
A1	Incline Press Machine (light weights)	2	10-12	2010	90 sec
A2	Prone Incline 2-Arm DB Row (light weights)	2	10-12	2010	90 sec
B1	Lean-Away DB Lateral Raise (light weights)	1	8-10	3011	10 sec
B2	Low Pulley Rope Curl (light weights)	1	8-10	30X0	10 sec
B3	EZ Bar Triceps Extension (light weights)	1	8-10	30X1	60 sec

Quads and Calves Unloading Workout (Hamstrings and Abs Touch-Up)

ORDER	EXERCISE	SETS	REPS	TEMPO	REST
A1	Heels Elevated DB Squat	2	10-12	2010	90 sec
A2	Standing Calf Raise Machine (light weights)	2	10-12	2010	90 sec
B1	Med-Ball or Weight Plate V-Up (light weights)	1	8-10	3011	10 sec
B2	Lying Leg Curl (light weights)	1	8-10	30X1	60 sec

Shoulders and Arms Unloading Workout (Chest and Back Touch-Up)

ORDER	EXERCISE	SETS	REPS	TEMPO	REST
A1	Seated DB Shoulder Press (light weights)	2	10-12	2010	60 sec
A2	Mid-Grip Straight Bar Scott Curl (light weights)	2	10-12	2010	60 sec
A3	EZ Bar Triceps Extension (light weights)	2	10-12	2010	60 sec
B1	Pec Deck Chest Fly	1	8-10	2012	10 sec
B2	DB Pullover on Flat Bench	1	8-10	3020	60 sec

Hamstrings and Abs Unloading Workout (Quads and Calves Touch-Up)

ORDER	EXERCISE	SETS	REPS	TEMPO	REST
A1	Lying Leg Curl (light weights)	2	10-12	2010	90 sec
A2	Med-Ball or Weight Plate V-Up (light weights)	2	10-12	2010	90 sec
B1	Standing Calf Raise Machine	1	8-10	1011	10 sec
B2	DB Bulgarian Split Squat (rear foot elevated)	1	8-10 ea	30X1	60 sec

Phase Three

Objective

For this phase, you will experience and stimulate all three mechanisms of muscle growth within the same workout! We will start with a mechanical tension-based exercise when you are still fresh. Then we'll move into a muscle damage exercise with a stretched position pause, which is great for creating soreness and stimulating growth. Finally, we'll finish off with some high rep exercises with short recovery to build up a lot of metabolites to help create cellular swelling (aka The PUMP!) and signal the muscles to grow.

Training Split

The recommended split for this phase is:

- Monday – Quads and Calves (Hamstrings Touch-Up)
- Tuesday – Chest and Abs (Back Touch-Up)
- Wednesday – Shoulders (Arms Touch-Up)
- Thursday – Hamstrings and Calves (Quads Touch-Up)
- Friday – Back and Abs (Chest Touch-Up)
- Saturday – Arms (Shoulders Touch-Up)
- Sunday – Off

Intensity Technique: *10+10+10 Drop Sets: Drop the weight 20 percent on each drop. However, if you cannot complete your 10 reps, continue to move the weight within the range that you still have available until you hit all 10 reps before reducing the weight to do the next drop. Continue to forcefully contract the muscle so that it burns like crazy. I don't care if the weight is only moving 2 inches. Do not put the weight down for even a second. Make it hurt!*

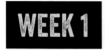

Workout One – Quads and Calves (Hamstrings Touch-Up)

ORDER	EXERCISE	SETS	REPS	TEMPO	REST
A	Barbell Back Squat	3	8	30X0	2-3 min
B	Alternating DB Drop Lunge	4	10 ea	41X0	90 sec
C	Leg Press	3	30	2010	60 sec
D	High Bench DB Step Ups (do all reps for 1 leg first)	3	30 ea	20X0	60 sec
E	Standing Calf Raise Machine	8	10	1011	20 sec
F	Standing Leg Curl	1	10+10+10 drop set*	30X1	N/A

*10+10+10 Drop Sets: *Review Intensity Technique on page 68.*

Workout Two – Chest and Abs (Back Touch-Up)

ORDER	EXERCISE	SETS	REPS	TEMPO	REST
A	Barbell Bench Press	3	8	30X0	2-3 min
B	Incline DB Chest Fly	4	10	41X0	90 sec
C	Incline DB Bench Press	3	30	2010	60 sec
D	Cable Crossover Chest Fly (high to low)	3	30	2011	60 sec
E	Swiss Ball Straight Leg Jackknife	3	10-15	2011	60 sec
F	Gironda Pulley Row	1	10+10+10 drop set*	30X1	N/A

*10+10+10 Drop Sets: *Review Intensity Technique on page 68.*

Workout Three – Shoulders (Arms Touch-Up)

ORDER	EXERCISE	SETS	REPS	TEMPO	REST
A	Mid-Grip Barbell Shoulder Press in Front	3	8	30X0	2-3 min
B	Lean-Away DB Lateral Raise	4	10 ea	41X0	90 sec
C	Bent Rear Delt Raise	3	30	2010	60 sec
D	DB Upright Row	3	30	2011	60 sec
E	Reverse Grip Triceps Pressdown with EZ Curl Attachment	1	10+10+10 drop set*	30X1	N/A
F	Low Pulley EZ Bar Curl	1	10+10+10 drop set*	30X1	N/A

*10+10+10 Drop Sets: *Review Intensity Technique on page 68.*

Workout Four – Hamstrings and Calves (Quads Touch-Up)

ORDER	EXERCISE	SETS	REPS	TEMPO	REST
A	Clean Grip Deadlift	3	7	30X0	2–3 min
B	DB RDL	4	10	41X0	90 sec
C	45-Degree Back Extension	3	30	2011	60 sec
D	Lying Leg Curl	3	30	20X0	60 sec
E	Seated Calf Raise (toes neutral)	5	15	1011	20 sec
F	Toe Press (calf raise on leg press machine)	5	10	1010	20 sec
G	Alternating Barbell Lunge	1	10+10+10 drop set* ea leg	20X0	N/A

*10+10+10 Drop Sets: *Review Intensity Technique on page 68.*

Workout Five – Back and Abs (Chest Touch-Up)

ORDER	EXERCISE	SETS	REPS	TEMPO	REST
A	Narrow Grip Neutral Chin-Up	3	7	30X0	2–3 min
B	Low Pulley 1-Arm Row from Lunge Position	4	10 ea	41X0	90 sec
C	1-Arm Neutral Grip Lat Pulldown	3	30 ea	2011	60 sec
D	Seated Cable Face Pull with Rope	3	30	2011	60 sec
E	Reverse Crunch with Med-Ball Between Knees	3	Max reps	1011	10 sec
F	Swiss Ball Rollouts from Knees	3	Max reps	3020	60 sec
G	Incline Barbell Bench Press	1	10+10+10 drop set*	30X0	N/A

*10+10+10 Drop Sets: *Review Intensity Technique on page 68.*

Workout Six – Arms (Shoulders Touch-Up)

ORDER	EXERCISE	SETS	REPS	TEMPO	REST
A1	Dips (torso upright)	3	7	30X0	90 sec
A2	Standing Barbell Curl	3	7	30X0	90 sec
B1	Incline DB Triceps Extensions	4	10	41X0	75 sec
B2	Incline DB Zottman Curl	4	10	41X0	75 sec
C1	Low Pulley Triceps Kickback (palm facing the ceiling in contracted position)	3	30 ea	2011	30 sec
C2	Prone Incline EZ Bar Spider Curl	3	30	2011	30 sec
D1	EZ Bar Triceps Extension	3	30	2110	30 sec
D2	Kneeling Dual High Pulley Curl	3	30	2011	30 sec
E	Rear Delt Cable Fly (high to low)	1	10+10+10 drop set*	30X0	N/A

*10+10+10 Drop Sets: *Review Intensity Technique on page 68.*

WEEK 6

Workout One - Quads and Calves (Hamstrings Touch-Up)

ORDER	EXERCISE	SETS	REPS	TEMPO	REST
A	Barbell Back Squat	5	3	30X0	2-3 min
B	Alternating DB Drop Lunge	4	8 ea	42X0	90 sec
C	Leg Press	3	20	2010	45 sec
D	High Bench DB Step Ups (do all reps for 1 leg first)	3	20 ea	20X0	45 sec
E	Leg Extension	3	20	2011	45 sec
F	Standing Calf Raise Machine	8	8	1011	20 sec
G	Standing Leg Curl	2	15	30X1	45 sec

Workout Two - Chest and Abs (Back Touch-Up)

ORDER	EXERCISE	SETS	REPS	TEMPO	REST
A	Barbell Bench Press	5	3	30X0	2-3 min
B	Incline DB Chest Fly	4	8	42X0	90 sec
C	Incline Barbell Bench Press	3	20	2010	45 sec
D	Cable Crossover Chest Fly (high to low)	3	20	2011	45 sec
E	Push-Up	3	20	2010	45 sec
F	Swiss Ball Straight Leg Jackknife	3	15-20	2011	60 sec
G	Gironda Pulley Row	2	15	30X1	45 sec

Workout Three - Shoulders (Arms Touch-Up)

ORDER	EXERCISE	SETS	REPS	TEMPO	REST
A	Mid-Grip Barbell Shoulder Press in Front	5	3	30X0	2-3 min
B	Lean-Away DB Lateral Raise	4	8 ea	42X0	90 sec
C	Bent Rear Delt Raise	3	20	2010	45 sec
D	DB Upright Row	3	20	2011	45 sec
E	Standing DB Lateral Raise	3	20	2011	45 sec
F	Reverse Grip Triceps Pressdown with EZ Curl Attachment	2	15	30X1	45 sec
G	Low Pulley EZ Bar Curl	2	15	30X1	45 sec

Workout Four – Hamstrings and Calves (Quads Touch-Up)

ORDER	EXERCISE	SETS	REPS	TEMPO	REST
A	Clean Grip Deadlift	5	3	30X0	2-3 min
B	DB RDL	4	8	42X0	90 sec
C	45-Degree Back Extension	3	20	2011	45 sec
D	Lying Leg Curl	3	20	20X0	45 sec
E	Low Pulley Pull Through	3	20	2010	45 sec
F	Seated Calf Raise (toes neutral)	5	12	1011	20 sec
G	Toe Press (calf raise on leg press machine)	5	8	1010	20 sec
H	Alternating Barbell Lunge	2	15 ea	20X0	45 sec

Workout Five – Back and Abs (Chest Touch-Up)

ORDER	EXERCISE	SETS	REPS	TEMPO	REST
A	Narrow Grip Neutral Chin-Up	5	3	30X0	2-3 min
B	Low Pulley 1-Arm Row from Lunge Position	4	8 ea	42X0	90 sec
C	1-Arm Neutral Grip Lat Pulldown	3	20 ea	2011	45 sec
D	Seated Cable Face Pull with Rope	3	20	2011	45 sec
E	Prone Incline 2-Arm DB Row	3	20	2010	45 sec
F	Reverse Crunch with Med-Ball Between Knees	3	Max reps	1011	10 sec
G	Swiss Ball Rollouts from Knees	3	Max reps	3020	60 sec
H	Incline Barbell Bench Press	2	15	30X0	45 sec

Workout Six – Arms (Shoulders Touch-Up)

ORDER	EXERCISE	SETS	REPS	TEMPO	REST
A1	Dips (torso upright)	5	3	30X0	90 sec
A2	Standing Barbell Curl	5	3	30X0	90 sec
B1	Incline DB Triceps Extensions	4	8	42X0	75 sec
B2	Incline DB Zottman Curl	4	8	42X0	75 sec
C1	Low Pulley Triceps Kickback (palm facing the ceiling in contracted position)	3	20 ea	2011	20 sec
C2	Prone Incline EZ Bar Spider Curl	3	20	2011	20 sec
D1	EZ Bar Triceps Extension	3	20	2110	20 sec
D2	Kneeling Dual High Pulley Curl	3	20	2011	20 sec
E1	Triceps Pressdown with Rope	3	20	2010	20 sec
E2	Low Pulley Rope Curl	3	20	2010	20 sec
F	Rear Delt Cable Fly (high to low)	2	15	2011	45 sec

WEEK 7

In weeks 7 to 9, for your tension workouts, you will be doing pyramids. For example, in week 7, it says 4 sets and the reps say 7,6,5,4. This means that you'll do *one* set of 7 reps, increase the weight and do one set of 6 reps, etc., until you've done 4 sets. Also, for the final weeks of this program, you will do the metabolic stress portions of the workout as giant sets and tri-sets. If you can't do this due to gym set-up, then simply do straight sets with 30 to 45 seconds rest.

Workout One – Quads and Calves (Hamstrings Touch-Up)

ORDER	EXERCISE	SETS	REPS	TEMPO	REST
A	Barbell Back Squat	4	7,6,5,4	30X0	2–3 min
B	Alternating DB Drop Lunge	5	6 ea	33X0	90 sec
C1	Leg Press	4	15	2010	10 sec
C2	High Bench DB Step Ups (do all reps for 1 leg first)	4	15 ea	20X0	10 sec
C3	Leg Extension	4	15	2011	75 sec
D	Standing Calf Raise Machine	6	20	1011	20 sec
E	Standing Leg Curl	3	12	30X1	45 sec

Workout Two – Chest and Abs (Back Touch-Up)

ORDER	EXERCISE	SETS	REPS	TEMPO	REST
A	Barbell Bench Press	4	7,6,5,4	30X0	2–3 min
B	Incline DB Chest Fly	5	6	33X0	90 sec
C1	Incline Barbell Bench Press	4	15	2010	10 sec
C2	Cable Crossover Chest Fly (high to low)	4	15	2011	10 sec
C3	Push-Up	4	15	2010	75 sec
D	Swiss Ball Straight Leg Jackknife	3	20–25	2011	60 sec
E	Gironda Pulley Row	3	12	30X1	45 sec

Workout Three – Shoulders (Arms Touch-Up)

ORDER	EXERCISE	SETS	REPS	TEMPO	REST
A	Mid-Grip Barbell Shoulder Press in Front	4	7,6,5,4	30X0	2–3 min
B	Lean-Away DB Lateral Raise	5	6 ea	33X0	90 sec
C1	Bent Rear Delt Raise	4	15	2010	10 sec
C2	DB Upright Row	4	15	2011	10 sec
C3	Standing DB Lateral Raise	4	15	2010	75 sec

CONTINUED

Workout Three - Shoulders (Arms Touch-Up)

ORDER	EXERCISE	SETS	REPS	TEMPO	REST
A	Mid-Grip Barbell Shoulder Press in Front	5	6,5,4,3,2	30X0	2-3 min
B	Lean-Away DB Lateral Raise	5	6 ea	33X0	90 sec
C1	Bent Rear Delt Raise	4	15	2010	10 sec
C2	DB Upright Row	4	15	2011	10 sec
C3	Standing DB Lateral Raise	4	15	2010	75 sec
D	Reverse Grip Triceps Pressdown with EZ Curl Attachment	3	12	2011	45 sec
E	Low Pulley EZ Bar Curl	3	12	30X1	45 sec

Workout Four - Hamstrings and Calves (Quads Touch-Up)

ORDER	EXERCISE	SETS	REPS	TEMPO	REST
A	Clean Grip Deadlift	5	6,5,4,3,2	30X0	2-3 min
B	DB RDL	5	6	33X0	90 sec
C1	45-Degree Back Extension	4	15	2011	10 sec
C2	Lying Leg Curl	4	15	20X0	10 sec
C3	Low Pulley Pull Through	4	15	2010	75 sec
D	Seated Calf Raise (toes neutral)	4	30	1011	20 sec
E	Toe Press (calf raise on leg press machine)	4	15	1010	20 sec
F	Alternating Barbell Lunge	3	12 ea	20X0	45 sec

Workout Five - Back and Abs (Chest Touch-Up)

ORDER	EXERCISE	SETS	REPS	TEMPO	REST
A	Narrow Grip Neutral Chin-Up	5	6,5,4,3,2	30X0	2-3 min
B	Low Pulley 1-Arm Row from Lunge Position	5	6 ea	33X0	90 sec
C1	1-Arm Neutral Grip Lat Pulldown	4	15 ea	2011	10 sec
C2	Seated Cable Face Pull with Rope	4	15	2011	10 sec
C3	Prone Incline 2-Arm DB Row	4	15	2010	75 sec
D	Reverse Crunch with Med-Ball Between Knees	3	Max reps	1011	10 sec
E	Swiss Ball Rollouts from Knees	3	Max reps	3020	60 sec
F	Incline Barbell Bench Press	3	12	30X0	45 sec

Workout Six - Arms (Shoulders Touch-Up)

ORDER	EXERCISE	SETS	REPS	TEMPO	REST
A1	Dips (torso upright)	5	6,5,4,3,2	30X0	90 sec
A2	Standing Barbell Curl	4	7,6,5,4	30X0	90 sec
B1	Incline DB Triceps Extensions	5	6	33X0	75 sec
B2	Incline DB Zottman Curl	5	6	33X0	75 sec
C1	Low Pulley Triceps Kickback (palm facing the ceiling in contracted position)	4	15 ea	2011	10 sec
C2	Prone Incline EZ Bar Spider Curl	4	15	2011	10 sec
C3	EZ Bar Triceps Extension	4	15	2110	10 sec
C4	Kneeling Dual High Pulley Curl	4	15	2011	10 sec
C5	Triceps Pressdown with Rope	4	15	2010	10 sec
C6	Low Pulley Rope Curl	4	15	2010	90 sec
D	Rear Delt Cable Fly (high to low)	3	12	2011	45 sec

WEEK 9

In weeks 7 to 9, for your tension workouts, you will be doing pyramids. For example, in Week 9, it says five sets and the reps say 5,4,3,2,1. This means that you'll do ONE set of 5 reps, increase the weight and do ONE set of 4 reps, etc., until you've done five sets. Also, for the final weeks of this program, you will do the metabolic stress portions of the workout as giant sets and tri-sets. If you can't do this due to gym set-up, then simply do straight sets with 30-45 seconds rest.

Workout One - Quads and Calves (Hamstrings Touch-Up)

ORDER	EXERCISE	SETS	REPS	TEMPO	REST
A	Barbell Back Squat	5	5,4,3,2,1	30X0	2-3 min
B	Alternating DB Drop Lunge	5	6 ea	33X0	90 sec
C1	Leg Press	4	15	2010	10 sec
C2	High Bench DB Step Ups (do all reps for 1 leg first)	4	15 ea	20X0	10 sec
C3	Leg Extension	4	15	2011	75 sec
D	Standing Calf Raise Machine	6	20	1011	20 sec
E	Standing Leg Curl	3	12	30X1	45 sec

Workout Two - Chest and Abs (Back Touch-Up)

ORDER	EXERCISE	SETS	REPS	TEMPO	REST
A	Barbell Bench Press	5	5,4,3,2,1	30X0	2-3 min
B	Incline DB Chest Fly	5	6	33X0	90 sec
C1	Incline Barbell Bench Press	4	15	2010	10 sec
C2	Cable Crossover Chest Fly (high to low)	4	15	2011	10 sec
C3	Push-Up	4	15	2010	75 sec
D	Swiss Ball Straight Leg Jackknife	3	20-25	2011	60 sec
E	Gironda Pulley Row	3	12	30X1	45 sec

Workout Three - Shoulders (Arms Touch-Up)

ORDER	EXERCISE	SETS	REPS	TEMPO	REST
A	Mid-Grip Barbell Shoulder Press in Front	5	5,4,3,2,1	30X0	2-3 min
B	Lean-Away DB Lateral Raise	5	6 ea	33X0	90 sec
C1	Bent Rear Delt Raise	4	15	2010	10 sec
C2	DB Upright Row	4	15	2011	10 sec
C3	Standing DB Lateral Raise	4	15	2010	75 sec
D	Reverse Grip Triceps Pressdown with EZ Curl Attachment	3	12	2011	45 sec
E	Low Pulley EZ Bar Curl	3	12	30X1	45 sec

Workout Four - Hamstrings and Calves (Quads Touch-Up)

ORDER	EXERCISE	SETS	REPS	TEMPO	REST
A	Clean Grip Deadlift	5	5,4,3,2,1	30X0	2-3 min
B	DB RDL	5	6	33X0	90 sec
C1	45-Degree Back Extension	4	15	2011	10 sec
C2	Lying Leg Curl	4	15	20X0	10 sec
C3	Low Pulley Pull Through	4	15	2010	75 sec
D	Seated Calf Raise (toes neutral)	4	30	1011	20 sec
E	Toe Press (calf raise on leg press machine)	4	15	1010	20 sec
F	Alternating Barbell Lunge	3	12 ea	20X0	45 sec

Workout Five - Back and Abs (Chest Touch-Up)

ORDER	EXERCISE	SETS	REPS	TEMPO	REST
A	Narrow Grip Neutral Chin-Up	5	5,4,3,2,1	30X0	2-3 min
B	Low Pulley 1-Arm Row from Lunge Position	5	6ea	33X0	90 sec
C1	1-Arm Neutral Grip Lat Pulldown	4	15 ea	2011	10 sec

ORDER	EXERCISE	SETS	REPS	TEMPO	REST
C2	Seated Cable Face Pull with Rope	4	15	2011	10 sec
C3	Prone Incline 2-Arm DB Row	4	15	2010	75 sec
D	Reverse Crunch with Med-Ball Between Knees	3	Max reps	1011	10 sec
E	Swiss Ball Rollouts from Knees	3	Max reps	3020	60 sec
F	Incline Barbell Bench Press	3	12	30X0	45 sec

Workout Six – Arms (Shoulders Touch-Up)

ORDER	EXERCISE	SETS	REPS	TEMPO	REST
A1	Dips (torso upright)	5	5,4,3,2,1	30X0	90 sec
A2	Standing Barbell Curl	5	5,4,3,2,1	30X0	90 sec
B1	Incline DB Triceps Extensions	5	6	33X0	75 sec
B2	Incline DB Zottman Curl	5	6	33X0	75 sec
C1	Low Pulley Triceps Kickback (palm facing the ceiling in contracted position)	4	15 ea	2011	10 sec
C2	Prone Incline EZ Bar Spider Curl	4	15	2011	10 sec
C3	EZ Bar Triceps Extension	4	15	2110	10 sec
C4	Kneeling Dual High Pulley Curl	4	15	2011	10 sec
C5	Triceps Pressdown with Rope	4	15	2010	10 sec
C6	Low Pulley Rope Curl	4	15	2010	90 sec
D	Rear Delt Cable Fly (high to low)	3	12	2011	45 sec

WEEK 10 – UNLOADING WEEK

Workout One - Quads and Calves (Hamstrings Touch-Up)

ORDER	EXERCISE	SETS	REPS	TEMPO	REST
A	Barbell Back Squat (light weights)	2	10-12	2010	2-3 min
B	Leg Press (light weights)	2	10-12	2010	2-3 min
C	Standing Calf Raise Machine (light weights)	2	10-12	1011	60 sec
D	Standing Leg Curl (light weights)	1	12	3011	N/A

Workout Two - Chest and Abs (Back Touch-Up)

ORDER	EXERCISE	SETS	REPS	TEMPO	REST
A	Barbell Bench Press (light weights)	2	10-12	3010	2-3 min
B	Pec Deck Chest Fly (light weights)	2	10-12	2011	60 sec

CONTINUED

(CONTINUED)

ORDER	EXERCISE	SETS	REPS	TEMPO	REST
C	Swiss Ball Straight Leg Jackknife	2	10-12	2011	60 sec
D	Gironda Pulley Row (light weights)	1	12	3011	N/A

Workout Three – Shoulders (Arms Touch-Up)

ORDER	EXERCISE	SETS	REPS	TEMPO	REST
A	Mid-Grip Barbell Shoulder Press in Front (light weights)	2	10-12	3010	2-3 min
B	Seated 2-Arm DB Lateral Raise (light weights)	2	10-12	2010	60 sec
C	Reverse Grip Triceps Pressdown with EZ Curl Attachment (light weights)	1	12	2011	N/A
D	Low Pulley EZ Bar Curl (light weights)	1	12	3011	N/A

Workout Four – Hamstrings and Calves (Quads Touch-Up)

ORDER	EXERCISE	SETS	REPS	TEMPO	REST
A	Clean Grip Deadlift (light weights)	2	10-12	2010	2-3 min
B	Lying Leg Curl (light weights)	2	10-12	2010	60 sec
C	Seated Calf Raise (toes neutral, light weights)	2	10-12	1011	45 sec
D	Alternating Barbell Lunge (light weights)	1	12 ea	2010	N/A

Workout Five – Back and Abs (Chest Touch-Up)

ORDER	EXERCISE	SETS	REPS	TEMPO	REST
A	Narrow Grip Neutral Chin-Up (light weights)	2	10-12	2010	2-3 min
B	Seated Cable Face Pull with Rope (light weights)	2	10-12	2011	60 sec
C	Reverse Crunch with Med-Ball Between Knees (light Med-Ball)	2	10-12	1011	60 sec
D	Incline Barbell Bench Press (light weights)	1	12	30X0	45 sec

Workout Six – Arms (Shoulders Touch-Up)

ORDER	EXERCISE	SETS	REPS	TEMPO	REST
A1	Dips (torso upright) (light weights)	2	10-12	3010	90 sec
A2	Standing Barbell Curl (light weights)	2	10-12	3010	90 sec
B1	Triceps Pressdown with Rope (light weights)	2	10-12	2010	45 sec
B2	Low Pulley Rope Curl (light weights)	2	10-12	2010	45 sec
C	Rear Delt Cable Fly (high to low) (light weights)	1	12	2011	N/A

PART 7

The Exercise Execution Demonstration Guide: Don't Do Another Rep Without These Max Contraction Cues

It's not what you do; it's how you do it. It doesn't matter how much you lift or how many reps you do if they all suck. Most people learn to lift weights by watching videos and looking at pictures in magazines. But exercise happens with the force you create internally, including *what you think about* while you do the actual movement. If I were standing next to you, I wouldn't be giving you cues about what you can figure out by watching a video or looking at a picture. I'd be telling you *what to think* so that you *initiate the movement with the working muscle* and direct maximum tension into the targeted muscle and nowhere else..

Exercise happens with what you do internally, including what you think while you do the actual movement.*

Here are a few critical "max contraction cues" to help you generate the greatest amount of tension within the muscle so that you get a high return for your time in the gym. Review these over and over. It takes a long time to retrain a muscle and break old crappy movement patterns. Pay close attention. You will not find these cues anywhere else.

ABS – OTHER MOVEMENTS

Swiss Ball Straight Leg Jackknife

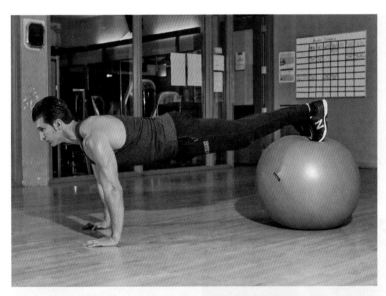

Cues:

- Don't let your hips move up and down— keep them in line with your shoulders.

- Bring your knees into your chest, flexing your lumbar spine, and squeeze your abs hard.

- Exhale all your air before reaching the top position to allow your abs to fully shorten.

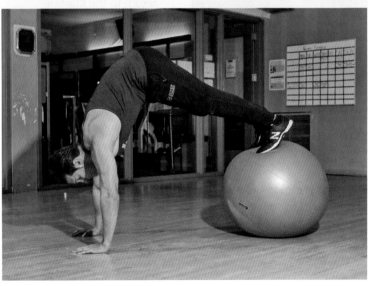

ABS – OTHER MOVEMENTS

Swiss Ball Rollouts from Knees

Cues:

- Lead with your hands, reaching out as far as you can while maintaining a neutral spine—avoid spinal extension.

- Contract your abs hard throughout to keep your pelvis neutral to ensure you challenge the abs and not the lower back.

- Don't allow your upper back and shoulders to round—keep your head, chest, and hips in a straight line.

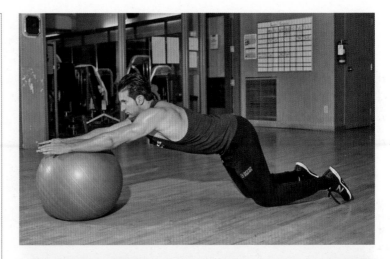

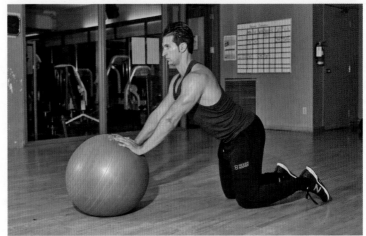

ABS – OTHER MOVEMENTS

Front Plank

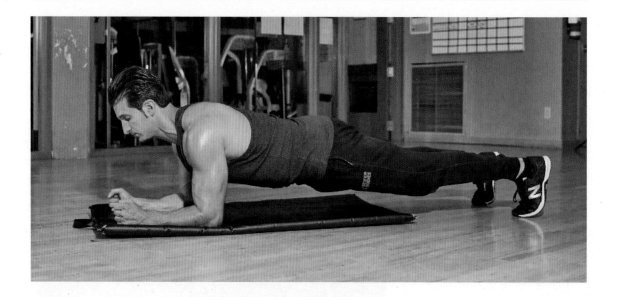

Cues:

■ Don't let your hips move up and down—keep them in line with your shoulders.

■ Don't allow your body to twist or tilt—keep your shoulders square.

■ Center your pelvis—it should not be tilted anteriorly or posteriorly. Think about driving your elbows and toes together to increase the contraction of your abs.

ABS – OTHER MOVEMENTS

Side Plank

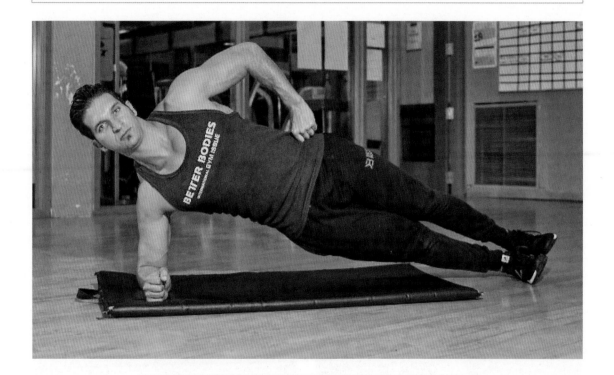

Cues:

- Don't let your hips move up and down—keep your body in a straight line.

- Don't allow your body to twist or tilt—keep your entire body perpendicular to the floor.

- Contract your abs, glutes, quads, and lats throughout.

ABS – OTHER MOVEMENTS

Wide Grip Palm Forward (overhand) Pull-Up

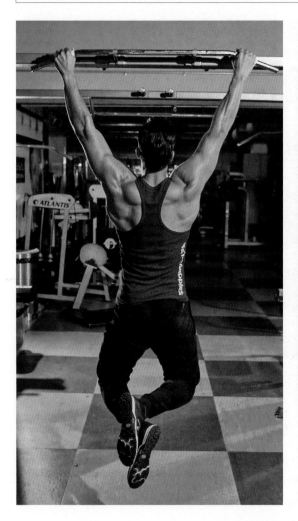 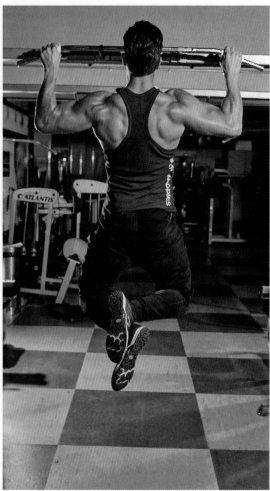

See cues on page 101

ABS – OTHER MOVEMENTS

Mid-Grip Supinated Pulldown

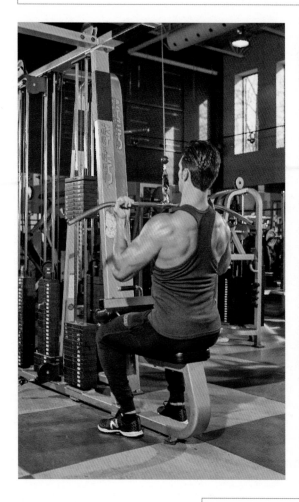 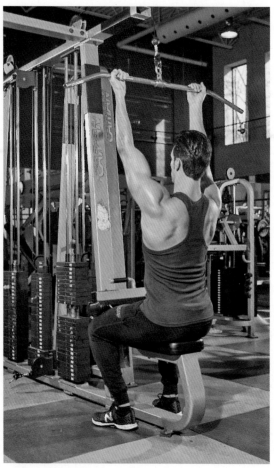

See cues on page 101

ABS – OTHER MOVEMENTS

Narrow Grip Neutral Chin-Up

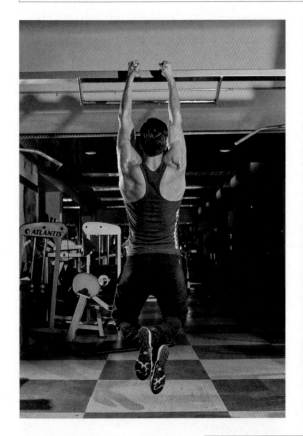
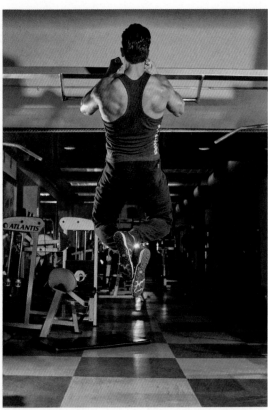

See cues on page 101

ABS – OTHER MOVEMENTS

1-Arm Neutral Grip Lat Pulldown

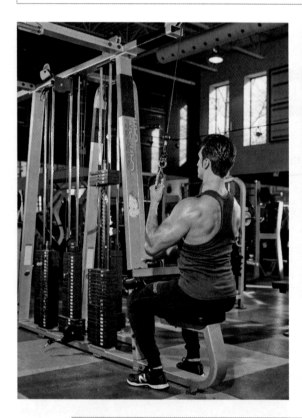 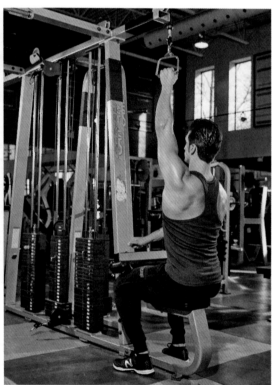

Cues

- Don't think about pulling down—think about pulling your elbows outward (pronated grip) or forward (supinated and neutral grips) in an arc.

- Don't think about pulling with your arms—retract and depress your shoulder blades as you pull to challenge the lats.

- Drive your elbows toward your lats (pronated grip) or behind you (supinated and neutral grips) to maximally shorten the lats.

BACK – OTHER MOVEMENTS

Seated Cable Face Pull with Rope

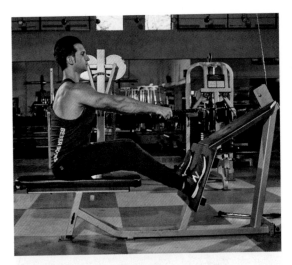 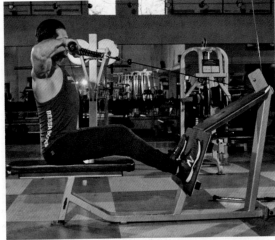

Cues:

■ Avoid any torso movement—keep your core braced and sit tall with your shoulders above your hips.

■ Don't think about pulling the rope toward you—think about ripping the rope apart and pulling your elbows out to opposite walls.

■ Don't let your elbows drop—keep your elbows slightly above your shoulders and pull the rope toward your nose.

BACK – OTHER MOVEMENTS

DB Pullover on Flat Bench

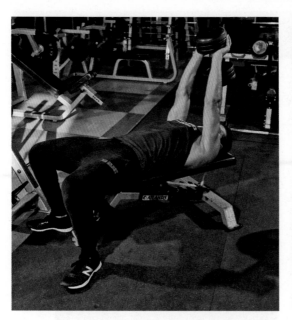 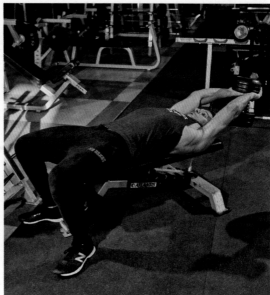

Cues:

■ Don't allow excessive spinal extension—brace your core and keep your lower back "locked down" to the bench.

■ Think about pushing the dumbbell as far away from you as possible and move the weight in an arc in both directions.

■ Don't think about moving the dumbbell up and down. Think about moving it backward and then forward.

BICEPS

BICEPS – ALL MOVEMENTS

Low-Pulley Rope Curl

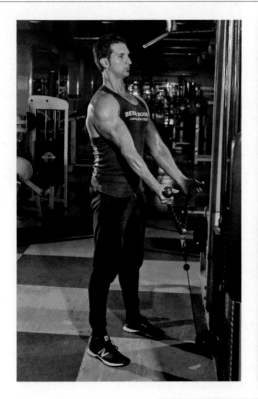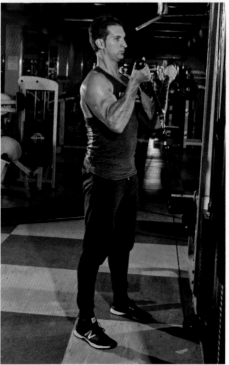

See cues on page 111

BICEPS – ALL MOVEMENTS

Low-Pulley EZ Bar Curl

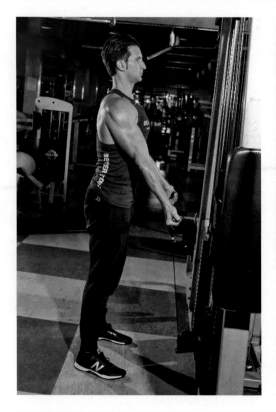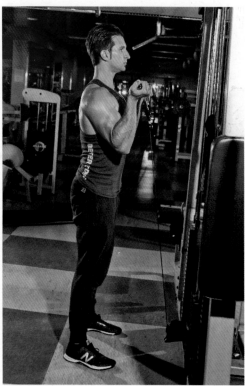

Cues:

- Don't think about curling the weight up—think about moving the weight forward for the first half of the rep and then backward for the second half of the rep, all while you concentrate on closing the gap between your forearm and biceps.

- Minimize movement of the upper arm—the majority of the movement should occur at the elbows, not the shoulder.

- Don't curl your wrists—keep them neutral or extend them slightly.

BICEPS – ALL MOVEMENTS

Kneeling Dual High Pulley Curl

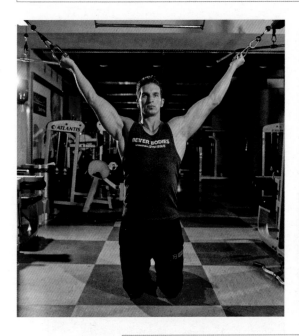 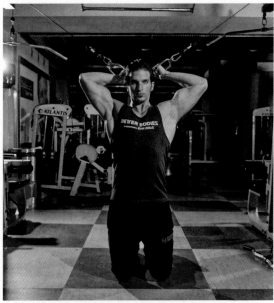

Cues:

■ Create some slight external rotation of your shoulder so that your biceps are facing upwards to begin.

■ Don't think about the cables in your hands. Think about closing the gap between your forearm and biceps.

■ Minimize movement from your upper arms and keep your body "locked down" the entire time.

BICEPS – ALL MOVEMENTS

Machine Curl

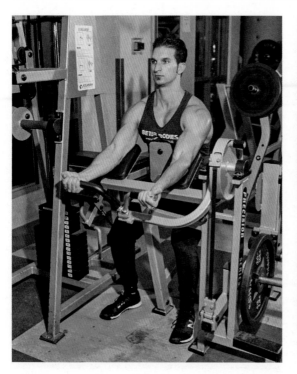 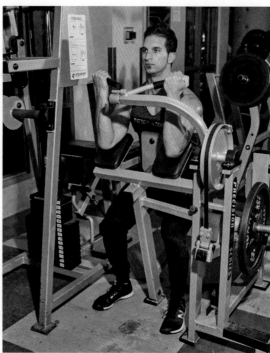

See cues on page 111

BICEPS – ALL MOVEMENTS

Prone Incline EZ Bar Spider Curl

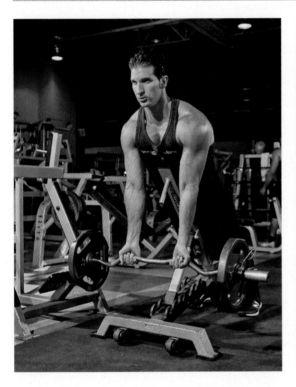 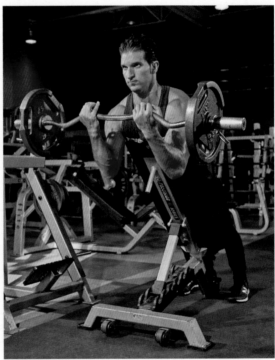

See cues on page 111

BICEPS – ALL MOVEMENTS

Incline DB Zottman Curl

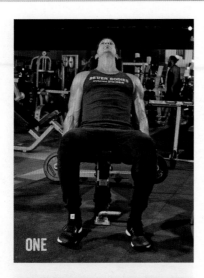
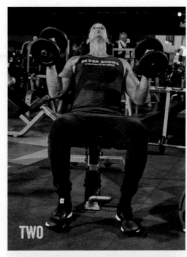
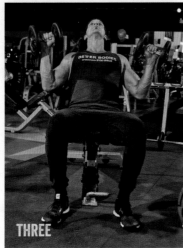
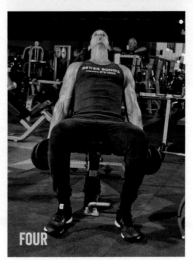

ONE

TWO

THREE

FOUR

See cues on page 111

BICEPS – ALL MOVEMENTS

Incline DB Hammer Curl

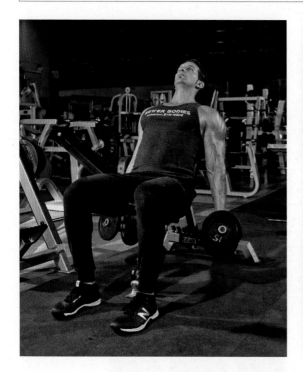 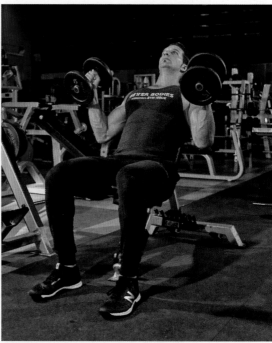

See cues on page 111

BICEPS – ALL MOVEMENTS

Incline DB Curl

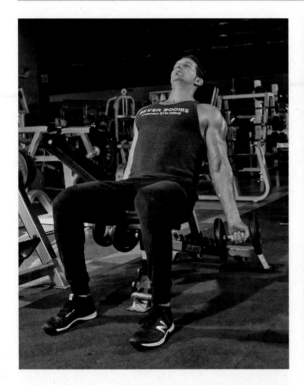 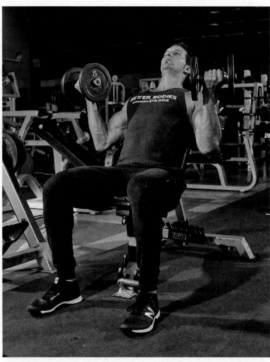

See cues on page 111

BICEPS – ALL MOVEMENTS

Standing DB Hammer Curl

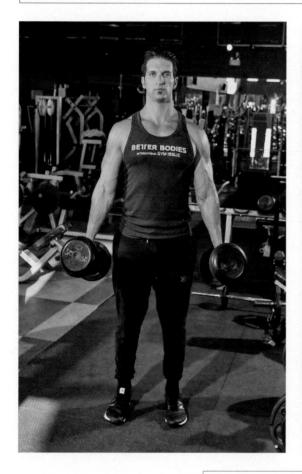 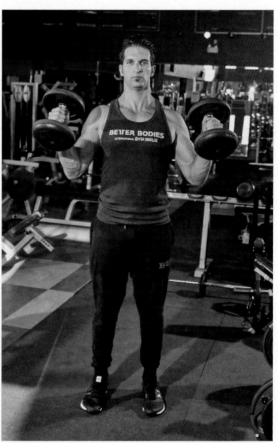

See cues on page 111

BICEPS – ALL MOVEMENTS

Standing Barbell Curl

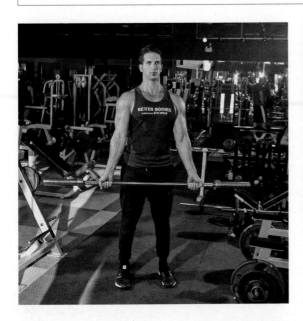 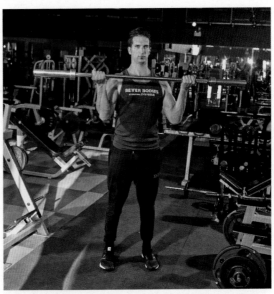

See cues on page 111

BICEPS – ALL MOVEMENTS

Standing Barbell Drag Curl

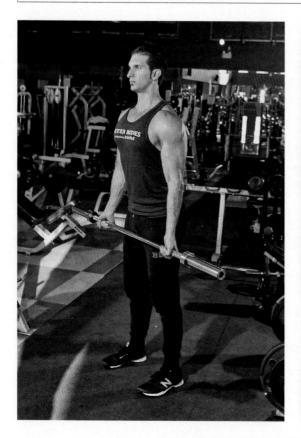 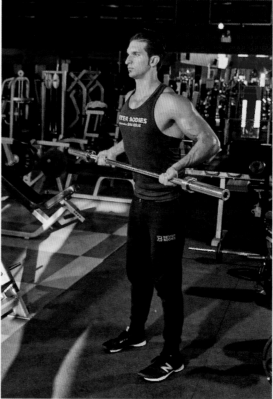

Cues:

■ Drag the bar up your body in a straight line while pulling your elbows backward until you experience a massive contraction.

■ Lower the bar in a straight line while letting your elbows move forward.

BICEPS – ALL MOVEMENTS

Mid-Grip Straight Bar Scott Curl

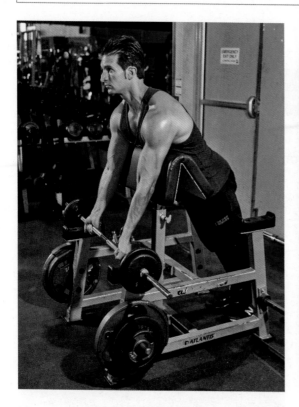 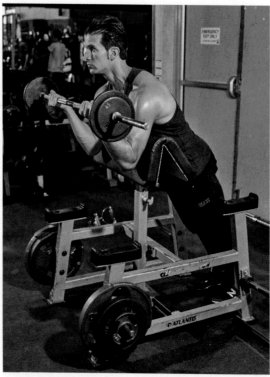

Cues:

- Drive your triceps into the pad before you initiate any contraction in the biceps and maintain constant contact the entire time.

- As you contract, close the imaginary line between your forearms and biceps. Think about your biceps crawling up and under your sleeve if you're wearing a t-shirt as you contract.

- At the top, reverse direction before your forearms become vertical to maintain constant tension on the biceps.

CALVES

CALVES – ALL MOVEMENTS

Toe Press (calf raise on leg press machine)

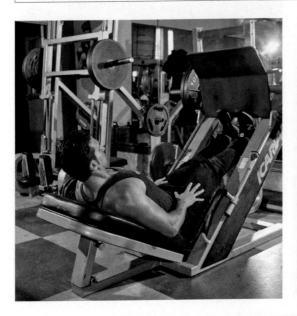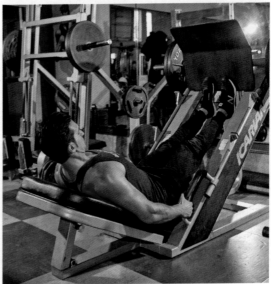

See cues on page 125

CALVES – ALL MOVEMENTS

Standing Calf Raise Machine

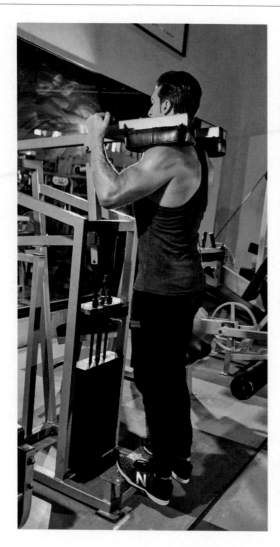
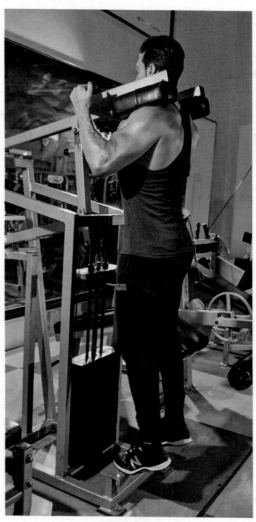

See cues on page 125

CALVES – ALL MOVEMENTS

Seated Calf Raise (toes neutral)

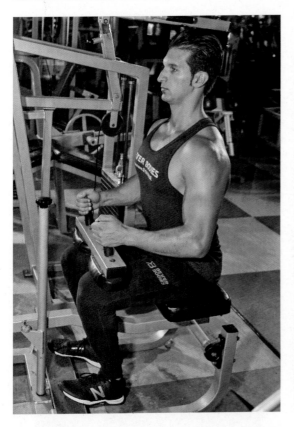 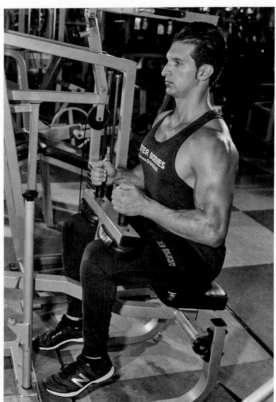

See cues on page 125

CALVES – ALL MOVEMENTS

Body Weight 1-Leg Calf Raise

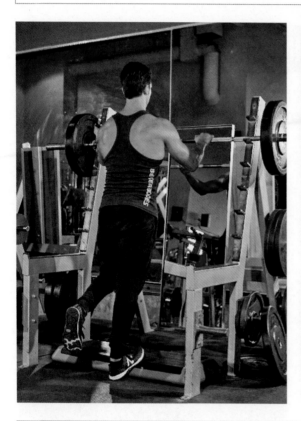 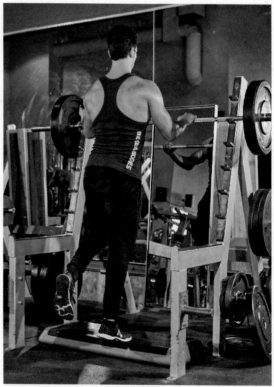

Cues:

■ Don't think about standing up—think about pushing your ankles forward to raise your heels as high as you can without rolling onto the outside of your feet.

■ Don't think about dropping down—think about pulling your ankles backward until you contract your anterior tibialis (muscle that runs along the shin) for a full stretch.

■ (Excluding Seated Calf Raises) Keep knees locked out and contract quads throughout so that you eliminate any assistance from your quads.

CHEST

CHEST – PRESSING MOVEMENTS

Barbell Bench Press

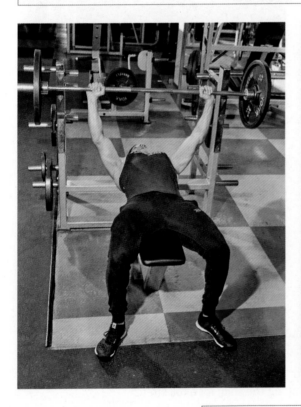
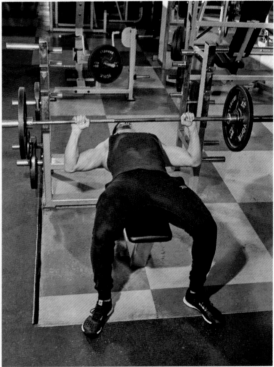

See cues on page 127

CHEST – PRESSING MOVEMENTS

Incline Barbell Bench Press

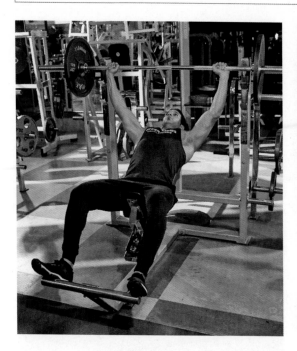 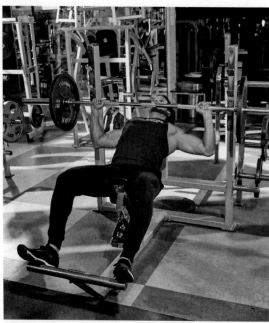

Cues:

- Don't think about pushing the weight up—think about pushing your elbows toward each other and across your body as you push your shoulders back into the bench.

- Keep your wrists directly above your elbows and finish each rep with your wrists slightly outside your shoulders.

- Don't just let the weight fall toward you—retract your shoulder blades and pull your elbows out and down.

CHEST – PRESSING MOVEMENTS

Incline DB Bench Press

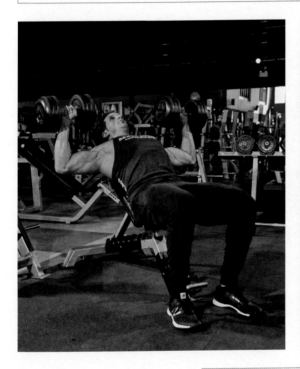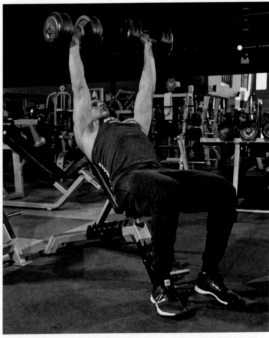

See cues on page 127

CHEST – PRESSING MOVEMENTS

Machine Chest Press

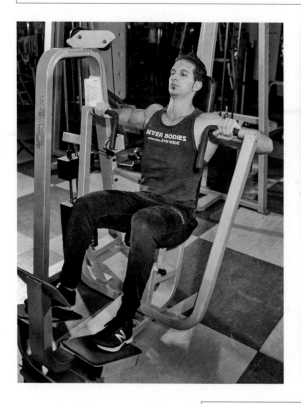 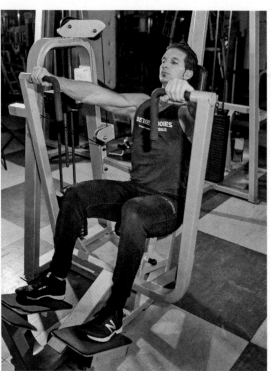

See cues on page 127

CHEST – PRESSING MOVEMENTS

Incline Press Machine

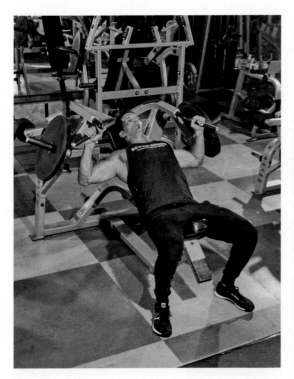 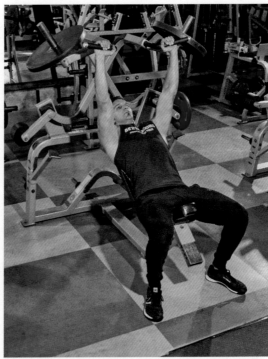

See cues on page 127

CHEST – PUSH-UPS

Push-Up

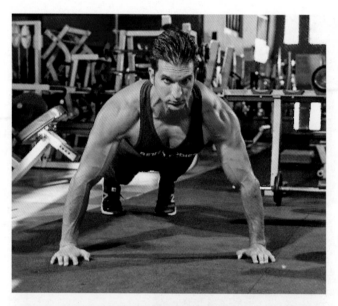

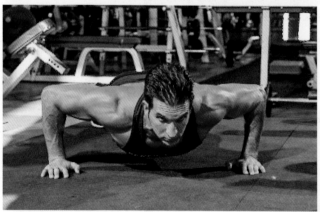

See cues on page 132

CHEST – PUSH-UPS

Shoulder Width Push-Up

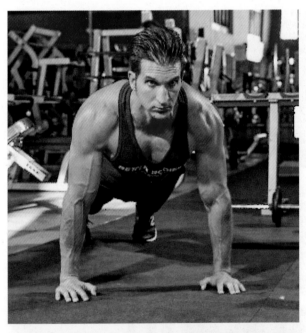

Cues:

- Don't think about pushing yourself up—think about pushing the floor away from you.

- Don't let your hips or lower back sag—contract your abs and glutes throughout to keep your body in a straight line.

- Don't just drop toward the ground— retract your shoulder blades and think about pulling yourself toward the floor.

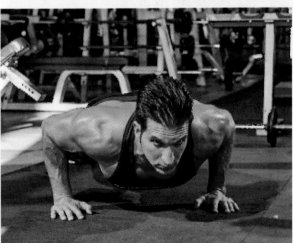

CHEST – FLY MOVEMENTS

DB Chest Fly

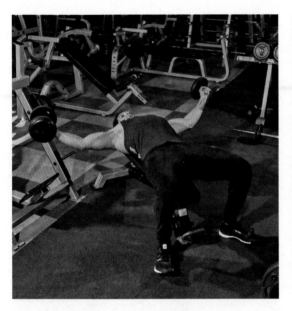 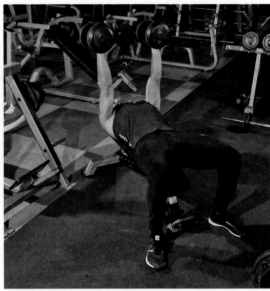

Cues:

- Don't let the weight pull you through the negative—retract your shoulder blades and pull your elbows out in an arc.

- Don't think about bringing your hands together—think about bringing your elbows together as you contract your pecs.

- With dumbbells, finish each rep with your wrists slightly outside your shoulders; with cables and machines, bring your elbows together as much as possible.

CHEST – FLY MOVEMENTS

Low Pulley Dual Cable Incline Fly

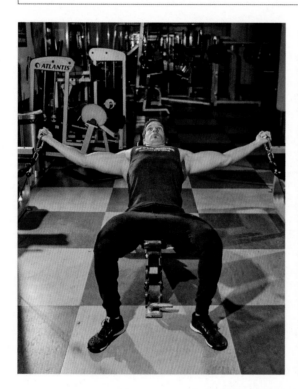 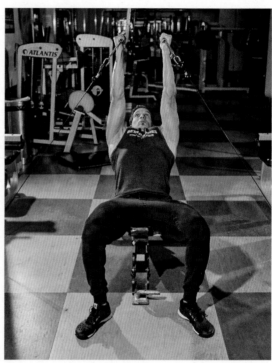

See cues on page 133

CHEST – FLY MOVEMENTS

Pec Deck Chest Fly

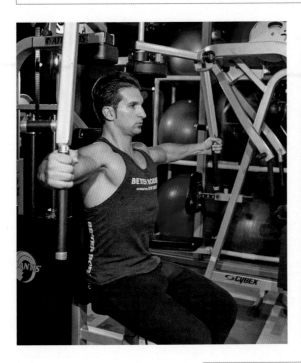 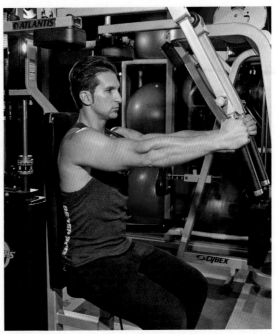

See cues on page 133

CHEST – FLY MOVEMENTS

Incline DB Chest Fly

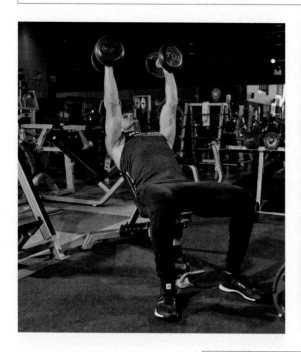 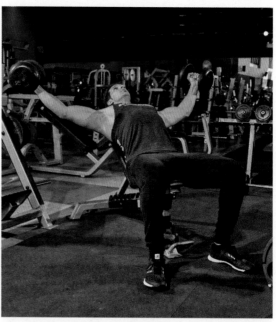

See cues on page 133

CHEST – FLY MOVEMENTS

Cable Crossover Chest Fly (high to low)

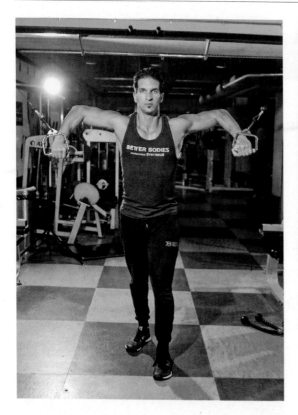 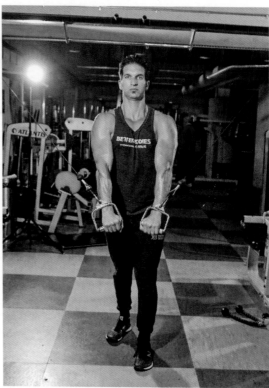

See cues on page 133

HAMSTRINGS

HAMSTRINGS – DEADLIFTS

Clean Grip Deadlift

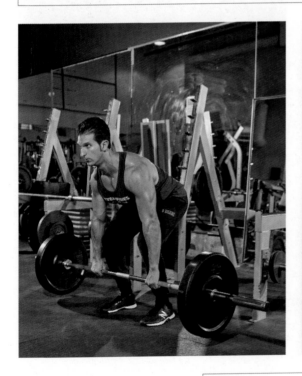 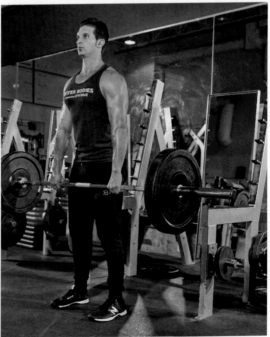

See cues on page 139

HAMSTRINGS – DEADLIFTS

Snatch Grip Deadlift

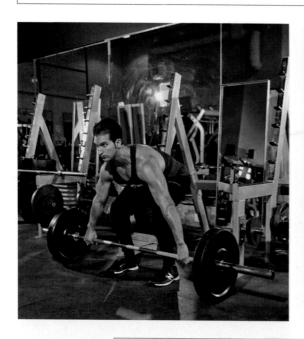 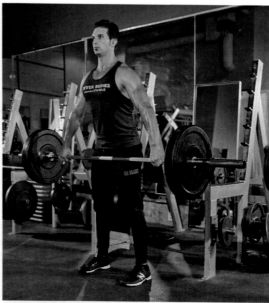

Cues:

■ Prior to the lift, pull a bend into the bar as you pull a slight arch into your lower back by pushing your hips back and pulling your chest tall.

■ Don't think about standing up—think about pushing the floor away from you and driving your hips forward.

■ Don't pull the bar with your upper body—keep your arms long and locked out and use your legs to move the weight.

HAMSTRINGS – STIFF-LEG MOVEMENTS

Low Pulley Pull Through

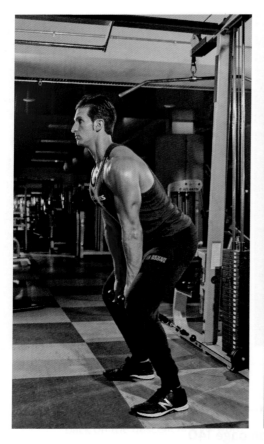 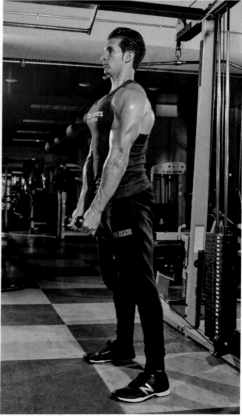

Cues:

- Don't "crowd" your groin—keep your arms long and locked out and reach back between your knees.

- Don't think about standing up and down, think about moving your hips back on the descent and forward on the ascent.

HAMSTRINGS – LEG CURLS

Lying Leg Curl

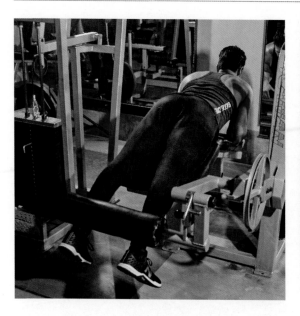 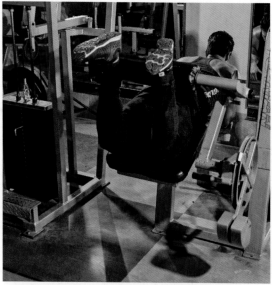

Cues:

- Don't let your hips move up and down, think about bracing your core and shoving your pelvis and hips into the pad throughout.

- Don't think about bringing your heels to your butt, think about closing the gap between your calves and your hamstrings.

- Avoid any torso movement—pretend your torso is stuck in cement.

HAMSTRINGS – LEG CURLS

Standing Leg Curl

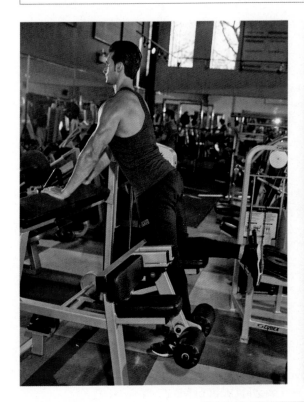 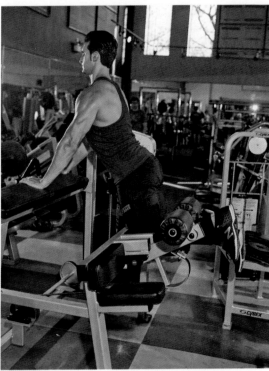

See cues on page 143

HAMSTRINGS – LEG CURLS

Swiss Ball Hip Bridge / Leg Curl Combo

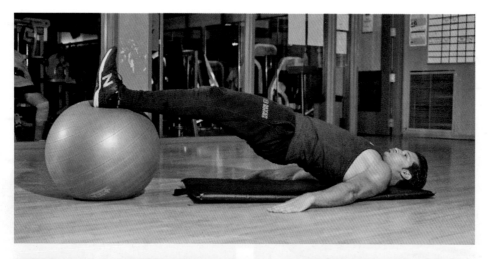

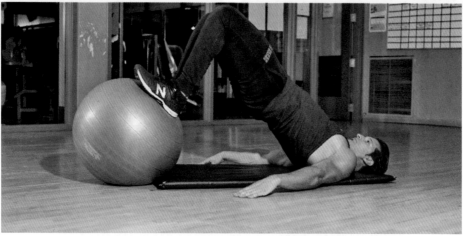

Cues:
- Drive your hips toward the ceiling as you close the gap between your calves and hamstrings.

QUADS

QUADS – SQUATTING MOVEMENTS

Barbell Back Squat

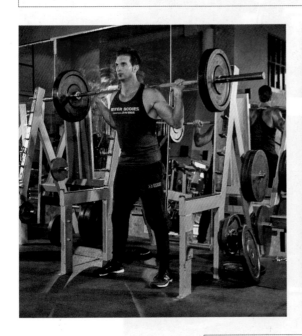 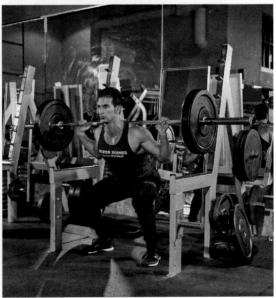

See cues on page 149

QUADS – SQUATTING MOVEMENTS

Heels Elevated Barbell Back Squat

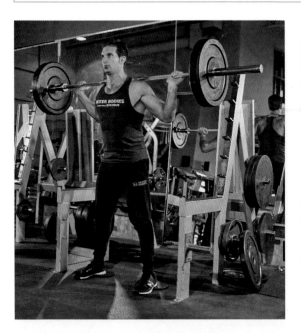 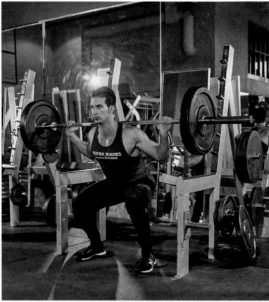

Cues:

■ On the descent, push your hips back and knees forward and slightly outward so that your knees track over your ankles; on the way up, push your hips forward and knees back.

■ Don't just drop down—shove your feet into the floor and think about pulling yourself down with your hamstrings.

■ Don't think about standing up—think about pushing the floor away from you.

QUADS – SQUATTING MOVEMENTS

Hack Squat Machine

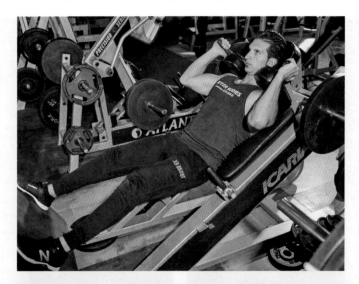

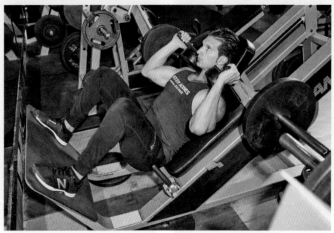

See cues on page 149

QUADS – LUNGES

Alternating DB Drop Lunge

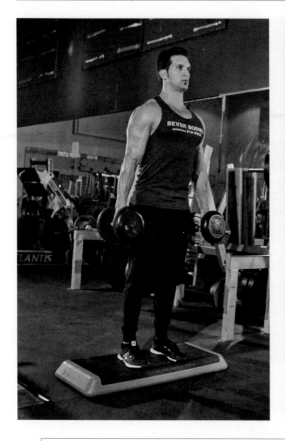 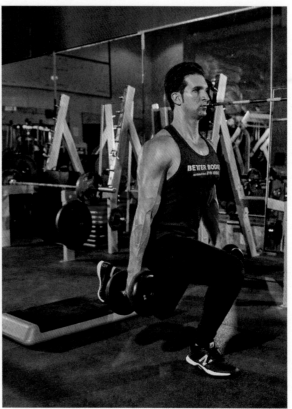

Cues:

- Don't think about standing up—think about pushing the floor away from you.
- Don't push with the front of your foot—push with the entire surface area of your foot.
- At the bottom, the angle of your shin should match that of your torso.

QUADS – LUNGES

Alternating Barbell Lunge

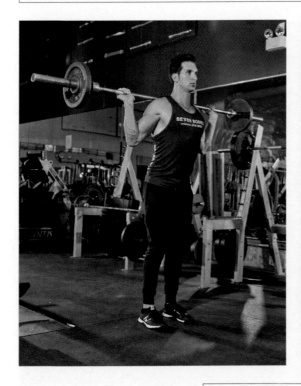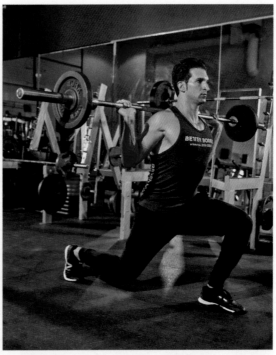

See cues on page 153

QUADS – STEP UPS AND DB BULGARIAN SPLIT SQUATS

DB Bulgarian Split Squat (rear foot elevated)

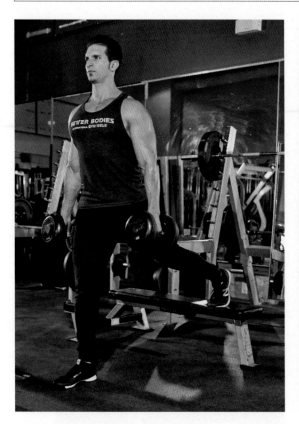
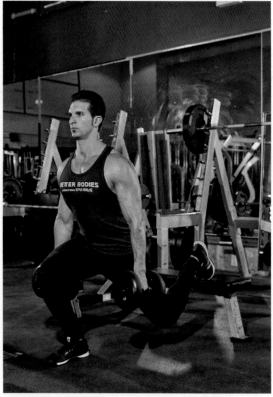

Cues:

- Don't use your back leg to assist—do all the work with your front leg.

- Don't push with the front of your foot—push with the entire surface area of your foot.

- At the bottom, the angle of your shin should match that of your torso.

QUADS — STEP UPS AND DB BULGARIAN SPLIT SQUATS

High Bench DB Step Ups

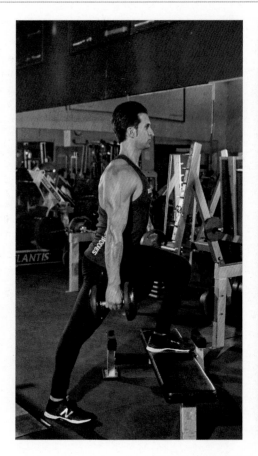 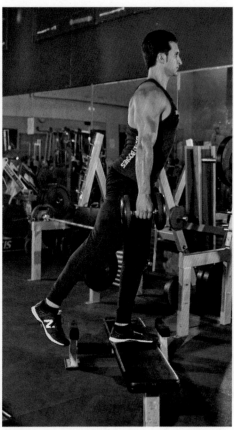

See cues on page 155

QUADS – LEG PRESS

Leg Press

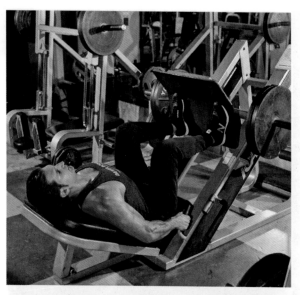

Cues:

- Don't just let the weight fall—pull your knees toward your chest.

- Don't allow your back to round at the bottom—maintain a slight arch to keep the tension in your legs, not your back. Use the handles to pull your butt into the seat.

- Don't allow any rotation at the hips—keep your hips, knees, and ankles in a straight line.

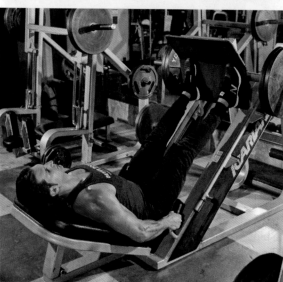

SHOULDERS – SIDE LATERAL MOVEMENTS

Prone Steep Incline DB Lateral Raise

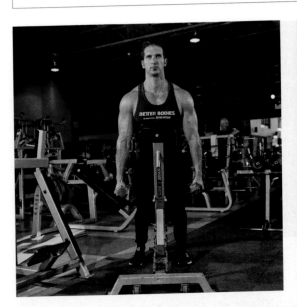 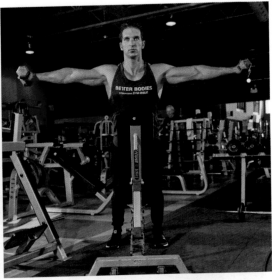

See cues on page 161

SHOULDERS – REAR DELT MOVEMENTS

Rear Delt on Pec Fly Machine

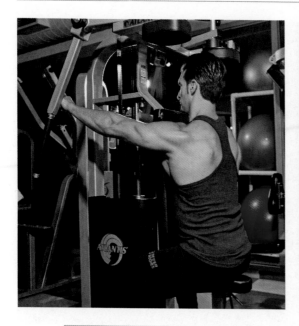 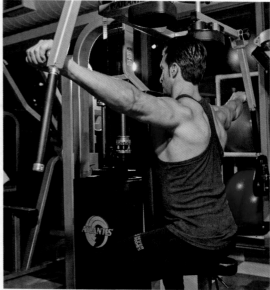

Cues:

■ Don't retract your shoulder blades—instead, protract your shoulders and think about keeping your hands as far away from you as possible and push your shoulders out and away throughout.

■ Don't think about pulling the weight backward—think about pushing the weight away from you and dragging your knuckles along the wall in front of you.

■ Reverse direction just before your shoulder blades start to retract to keep the tension in your rear delts and prevent assistance from the traps.

SHOULDERS – REAR DELT MOVEMENTS

Bent Rear Delt Raise

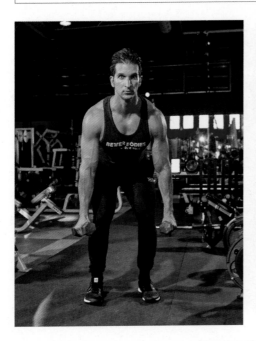 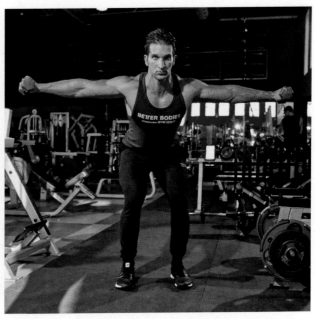

See cues on page 165

SHOULDERS – REAR DELT MOVEMENTS

Rear Delt Cable Fly (high to low)

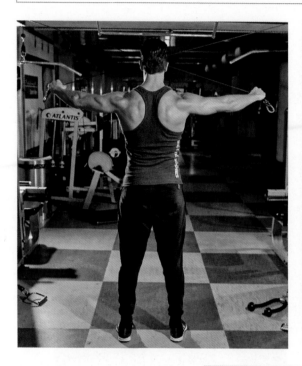 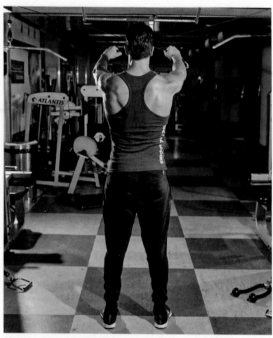

See cues on page 165

SHOULDERS – UPRIGHT ROWS

Snatch Grip Upright Row

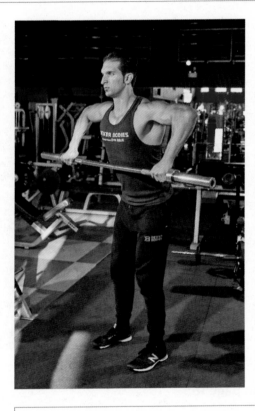 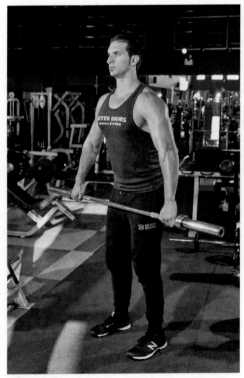

Cues:

■ Don't think about pulling the weight up—think about pulling your elbows out and away from you in an arc.

■ Reverse direction just before your forearms start to angle up toward the ceiling to keep the tension in your delts and prevent assistance from the forearms.

■ Don't just let the weight fall— retrace that same arc of the elbows on the negative (as you lower the weight) and maintain constant tension.

SHOULDERS – UPRIGHT ROWS

DB Upright Row

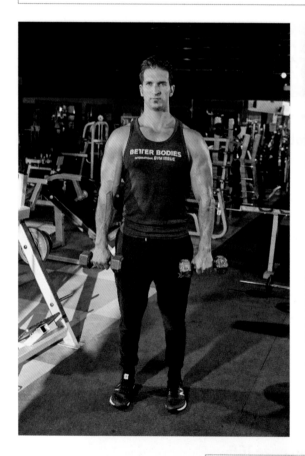
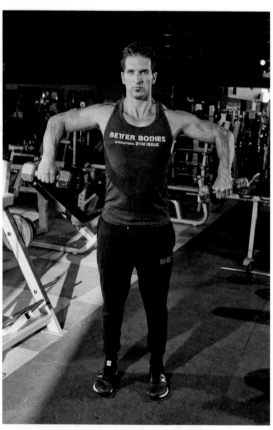

See cues on page 168

TRICEPS – EXTENSION MOVEMENTS

Triceps Extension Machine

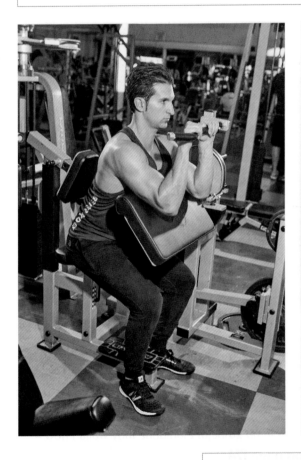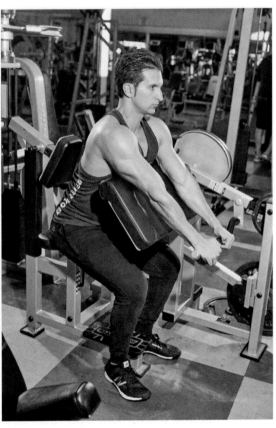

See cues on page 174

TRICEPS – EXTENSION MOVEMENTS

Seated EZ Bar French Press (overhead triceps extension)

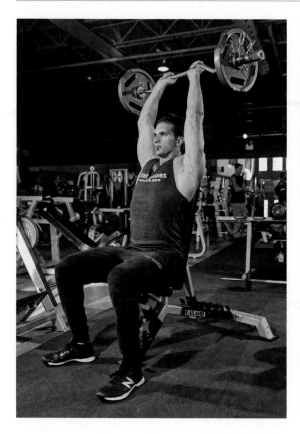
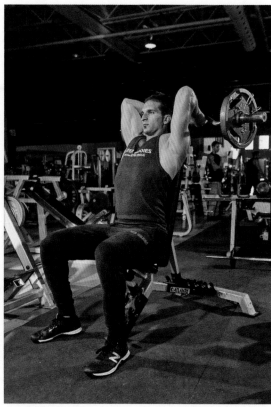

See cues on page 174

TRICEPS – EXTENSION MOVEMENTS

EZ Bar Triceps Extension

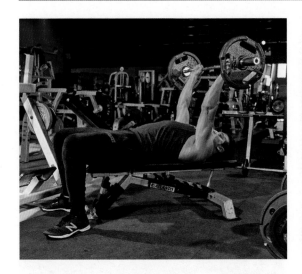 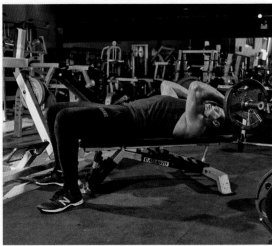

See cues on page 174

TRICEPS – EXTENSION MOVEMENTS

Dips (torso upright)

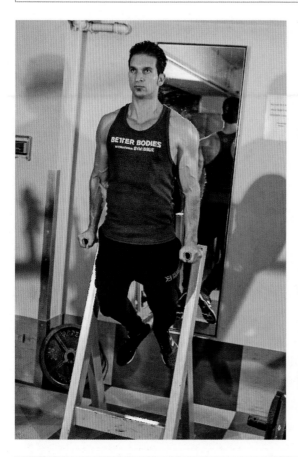
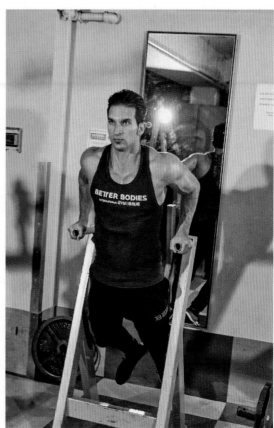

Cues:

- Don't think about pushing yourself up—think about pushing the bars away from you.
- Don't allow your elbows to flare out—maintain external rotation at the shoulder throughout.
- Don't allow your shoulders to shrug up or round forward—do your best to keep your shoulder blades retracted and depressed.

TRICEPS – EXTENSION MOVEMENTS

Close Grip Barbell Bench Press (shoulder width)

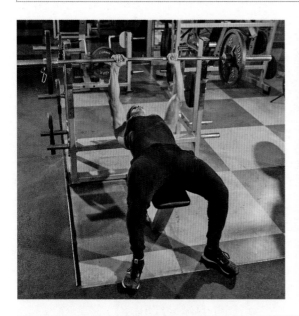 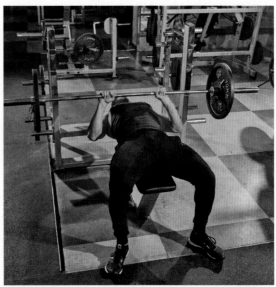

Cues:

- Don't think about pushing the weight up—think about pushing your elbows toward each other and across your body as you push your shoulders back into the bench.

- Don't think about squeezing your chest—focus on squeezing your triceps throughout.

- Don't tuck your elbows into your sides—keep your elbows outside of your hands.

PART 8

Five Rituals to Rapid Recovery

Increased muscle mass occurs because of *two* main causes—training *and recovery.*

One of the most important ideas I learned from Australian strength coach Ian King is: "Training in itself does not produce the training results."

He explained that the training session stimulates the change, but the actual changes can only be optimized when "training is matched with a suitable recovery."

If your training regimen exceeds your ability to recover, you will not achieve the training effect you desire. Suitable recovery includes time off between workouts and certain methods that assist the restorative process.

You are what you can recover from!

To sum up: *You are what you can recover from!* With this truth in mind, it only makes sense that your focus should be on taking the appropriate measures to ensure your body has everything it needs to recover. While there are thousands of recovery strategies out there, I'm going to share a few long-time favorites that have worked tremendously well for my clients and me. You don't have to apply all of them at the same time though.

Recovery Ritual #1: Contrast Baths and Showers

When I ran varsity cross-country at Western University, one of the strategies our team used to combat our heavy training volume was contrast baths and showers. The rate of recovery was noticeably different, and if it weren't I would have kicked this strategy to the curb. Trust me, I don't sit in 60 degree or colder water for fun!

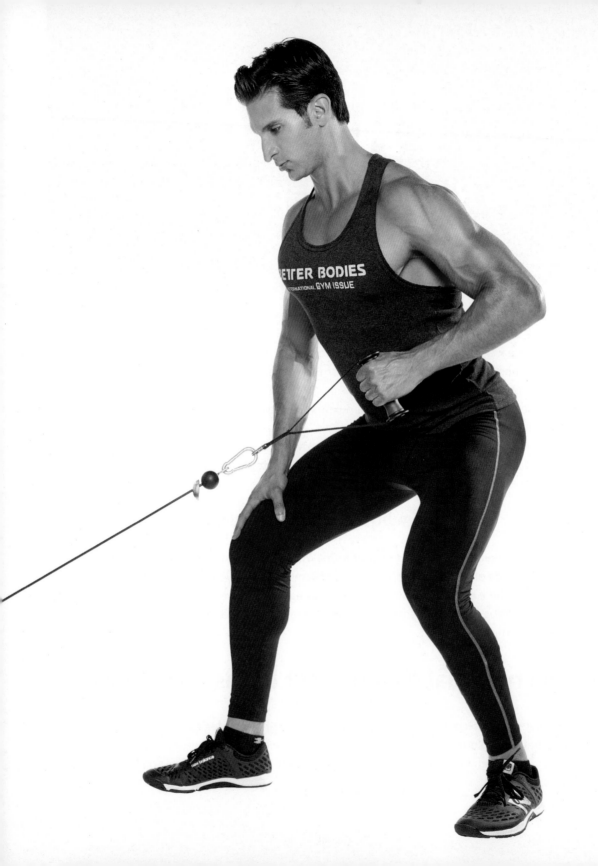

The optimal protocol is to alternate between 1 minute of cold water and 2 minutes of hot water for up to five rounds. This technique is very effective at increasing peripheral blood flow, thus facilitating recovery.[22]

The biggest advantage of contrast showers when it comes to building muscle is that it helps you remove a lot of the metabolic by-products of training—things that make you feel sore the next day, like lactate.[23]

Recovery Ritual #2: Massage

One of the best ongoing investments I make in my own training is massage therapy. Building muscle always relies on the health of your body's internal tissues, which requires optimal circulation of fresh blood, oxygen, and nutrients and the ability to remove toxins.[24] This can all be achieved with the varying types of strokes of a massage therapist.

Stretching the tissues during a massage helps muscle fibers release tension and pressure buildup. The massage helps stretch muscles both lengthwise and sideways along the natural blood flow across the muscle tissues. The following are some of the benefits associated with massage:

1) Greater flexibility[25]
2) Improved circulation[26]
3) Reduced pain[27]
4) Improved sleep[28]
5) Decreased tension[29]

I've found that getting a deep-tissue massage at least two times per month is optimal. During extremely intense training phases, you might consider going once per week. Or if that's not in the budget, be sure to get a massage at least once every 10 weeks. Your body will thank you with improved performance.

Recovery Ritual #3: Muscle Activation Technique (MAT™)

MAT has changed my life. If I could only prescribe one recovery ritual for the rest of my life this would be it. Every time I get a treatment, I feel like I'm walking out with an S on my chest. "Look out, here comes Superman!"

MAT is based on a very simple premise known as the Roskopf Principle,[30] which gets pretty scientific. But in simple terms, if you have a muscle that refuses to grow, then there is a very good chance it's not "turned on." It's unable to contract, leaving the muscle you're trying to train weak, and the opposing muscle tight.

When I first started seeing a MAT specialist, my body had muscle weaknesses everywhere. I was unable to sprint. In fact, any form of running left me crippled for days. I was constantly tight and didn't move fluidly. Leg training would leave my lower back sore for weeks. People told me this pain was simply because of how hard I trained. Others told me it was because I sit at my desk all day. Both camps were wrong. After working with Eric Seifert, my MAT specialist in Ontario, we were able to identify and treat my weak links. Now I'm able to sprint up to three times per week plus train my legs without being debilitated. My body also looks more balanced and my muscles contract more forcefully, which allows me to build muscle "easier." The best part about MAT is that a single session can stick for weeks. If you can't tell, I'm a raving disciple of the therapy. Thank God for Greg Roskopf and MAT!

Recovery Ritual #4: Handling Stress

The French eat baguettes, croissants, fatty meats, creamy sauces, and rich desserts, and drink lots of wine. They basically do everything health experts in North America tell us not to do, and yet *Forbes* magazine reported a 2014[31] comparison study of health in eleven industrialized nations, and France ranked number-one for healthy lives, while the U.S. ranked dead last.[32]

Why? We are far more stressed out than the French. Stress stimulates the body to produce cortisol, and too much cortisol will mess with your health and hinder your ability to lose fat or put on muscle.[33] To build 30 pounds of muscle in 30 weeks, you must keep cortisol levels under control.

One problem with stress is there are so many triggers coming at you each day, and it's impossible to control what hits when. Some sources include:

- Heavy traffic
- Your kid is in trouble at school
- Your girlfriend left you for your best friend
- The IRS is after you
- You lost your phone
- People are getting laid off at work, and you're wondering if you're next

The list goes on and on. Cortisol also can overload your system when you're exposed to pollution, junk food, overtraining, and too much caffeine, and also when you don't get enough sleep.

You can't control what happens to you, but you can learn to control how you respond. The best way to manage cortisol is to start adding these tools to your anti-stress toolbox:

- Script out tomorrow's day before you go to bed
- Go to bed 30 minutes early to get better sleep
- Spend at least 5 minutes praying or meditating when you rise
- Participate in yoga or stretch for anywhere from 15 to 60 minutes a day
- Kiss someone or tell someone how much you appreciate him or her

- Don't turn on your phone or look at your email until after lunch
- Stay hydrated and don't skip any of your planned meals
- Listen to inspirational podcasts while you're in your car
- Start outsourcing projects and "to dos" that you hate doing
- Hang out with people who have a positive outlook on life
- Indulge in a TV series that allows you to completely disconnect
- Have at least one date night per week with your partner or spouse and spend time with your friends and family at least once per week
- Plan a "No Screen Saturday" where you view zero screens for a day
- Have sex for as long and as often as possible
- Look at tests and trials as gifts and opportunities to grow
- Read at least one book per month
- Take a vacation as often as possible
- Surround your world with laughter
- Take a power nap
- And most important, as we Italians say, "*Fuhgeddaboudit*"

You can't control what happens to you, but you can learn to control how you respond.

Recovery Ritual #5: Sleep

Of all of the recovery strategies, this is by far the most important. Your body cannot function to its true potential without a restful night's sleep. Poor sleep will leave you more prone to putting on fat, slow your recovery, and impede gains in both strength and muscle mass. A lack of sleep will quickly wreak havoc on your hormone profile, including causing a drop in key recovery hormones such as testosterone and growth hormone. Other side effects are increased cortisol levels,[34] decreased thyroid function,[35] decreased motivation, increased craving for junk food,[36] compromised immune system,[37] increased chance of injury, and the list goes on.

Key to improving both the quantity and quality of your sleep is developing better bedtime habits. Teach your body when it's time to shut down for the night. After a few weeks of practice you'll notice a huge improvement in sleep quality—without pills or prescriptions.

Here are seven simple and actionable steps that you can begin immediately. Don't panic if you don't notice a change right away. Some people require a little longer for habit shifts to kick in.

Step 1: Hydrate throughout the day. Drink a minimum of a gallon (128 ounces or 3.75 liters) of water or 70 percent of your body weight in ounces per day. If you weigh 180 pounds, drink 126 ounces of pure water. If you've been sweating a lot, sprinkle in a little colored salt (such as Himalayan pink salt) to bring your electrolytes back into balance.[38]

Step 2: Make sure you get enough zinc and magnesium. These two minerals help your body slide into a good night's sleep.[39] If you buy a magnesium supplement, for best absorption, opt for magnesium gluconate, magnesium lactate, or magnesium citrate.[40]

Step 3: Establish a regular bedtime. Building better habits is a crucial part of improving sleep quality, and one of those habits is going to bed around the same time each and every night. When sleep becomes a part of a regular routine, then falling asleep on time becomes infinitely easier.

Step 4: Create the optimal sleep environment. To ensure a good night's sleep, at least one hour before you go to bed, unwind and unplug. Turn off the TV, put your cell phone away from your bed, and unplug all nearby electrical equipment (you may use a fan for white noise). If you set an alarm, use a cheap watch, as it has no electrical activity. Use a mask to block light when you travel, or if your bedroom never gets completely dark.[41] Also, keep the room cool. Room temperature should be 67 to 70 degrees. You will fall asleep faster and also get a more restful night's sleep in a colder environment.

Step 5: Clear your mind. A lot of people bring the anxiety of their day to bed with them, and that can make it hard to fall (or stay) asleep. The best solution is to clear your mind before you go to bed. Write down anything you're thinking about that you need to accomplish the next day. Doing this will eliminate the "I can't forget this" chatter that might keep you tossing and turning all night. Write these tasks down and release them from your mind, so your mind can relax and get ready for a restful sleep.

Step 6: Read before bed. I find that any type of book is great before bedtime, and after 5 to 30 minutes reading, I'm out cold! One important note: for the best rest, read old-fashioned print books. Lit screens reduce melatonin production and make it harder to fall asleep.[42]

Step 7: Use minimal light after 6 p.m. The body is light sensitive, and the presence of light signals "daytime," which leads to disruption of your body's internal clock and reduced production of melatonin. The more you are exposed to light in the evening, the less sleepy you'll be.[43]

To optimize sleep benefits, aim for seven to nine hours of sleep per night.[44] The best situation is to go to bed early enough so that your body wakes up naturally, without an alarm clock.

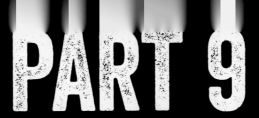

PART 9

Fourteen Simple, No-Nonsense Nutrition Principles to Gain Your First 30 Pounds of Pure Muscle

It seems everyone feels pressure to fit into a diet camp or nutrition cult these days—carb cycling, ketogenic, paleo, vegan, flexible dieting, and if you don't belong to one then you're the wacko! People's diets have become their identities, and my advice is: when someone tells you that you *must* eat one particular way, *run*! The best muscle-building results come when you *simplify* nutrition and don't complicate it with minutiae and nonsense. Trust sources that stick to the science and teach sustainable approaches that show how you can still enjoy your favorite foods while achieving your goals. In this section, we'll cover the simple, no-nonsense principles to gaining your first 30 pounds of pure muscle.

The Nutritional Hierarchy of Muscle Growth (and Fat Loss)

If you could ask me just one question about nutrition, what would it be? If your question has anything to do with supplements, you're majoring in the minors and maybe minoring in the majors. You're too focused on details that have marginal impact. You need to understand the big picture.

There is a specific order of importance when setting up your diet. If you don't understand the most impactful variables, you'll waste time and money.

I believe people are confused about what's important because the important variables are, frankly, boring, basic, and not at all sexy. But it's the nonsexy information that delivers the best results.

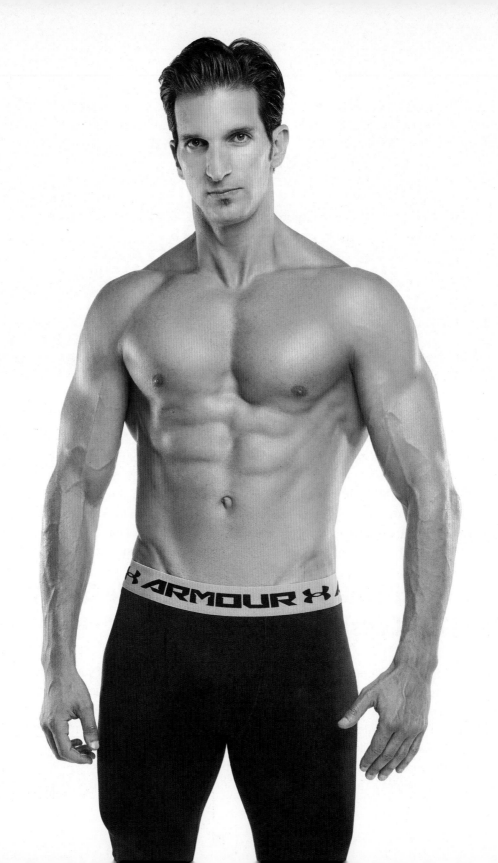

The least important variables, such as supplements and nutrient timing, are exciting and sexy! Sexy sells. Sexy goes viral. Sexy can confuse the heck out of you. Under the right conditions, you can incorporate the sexy variables, but first you must dial in all the basics.

First—calories. How many you take in versus how many you use will determine whether you gain, lose, or maintain weight. Surprisingly, this is the most neglected variable.

Second—macronutrients. How much protein, fat, carbs, fiber, and alcohol you consume will have the greatest impact on your body composition—which ratio of those calories get converted to muscle mass and/or fat.

Complicated is your enemy. Just handle your calories, then macros, and forget the other points until you master these two.

Third—micronutrients and hydration. If you are dehydrated, building muscle is nearly impossible, no matter how much creatine or other supplements you use. Stick to the meal plans, and you'll get sufficient fruits and vegetables to safeguard against deficiencies.

Nutrient timing and supplements are fourth and fifth respectively. They are only minor factors when you're going after your first 30 pounds of muscle, but I will say a little about each in parts 10 and 11.

My advice to you is the K.I.S.S. Principle: Keep It Simple, Stud-man!

Focus on simple, simple, simple. Complicated is your enemy. Just handle your calories, then macros, and forget the other points until you master these two.

Choose Your Goal:
Don't Chase Two Rabbits at Once

"If you chase two rabbits, both will escape."
—ANONYMOUS

You're either cutting (losing weight) or bulking (gaining weight). Beginners can sometimes achieve both for a brief period, but very few people dramatically transform their body when they pursue bulking up and getting lean at once. With a split focus, they don't achieve either one. Don't be that guy.

Focus on one goal and one goal only until you achieve it. Do not shift your focus until you accomplish the original goal. If you start out with 12 percent body fat or less, and your first goal is to build muscle, submerge your life in muscle and don't even give cutting a second thought until you achieve the muscle mass you desire.

When it comes time to get lean, apply the same laserlike focus. The end result will become dramatically bigger and leaner. Your friends won't recognize you.

Calories and Macronutrients: Setting Your Best Targets (Without Complicated Formulas)

Calories are the most important factor to body weight regulation (whether you want to build muscle or lose fat). You can have the perfect macros, nutrient timing, and meal frequency strategies in existence; you can have the highest quality supplements money can buy; you can avoid all the alcohol, gluten, and dairy in the world, but it won't mean squat if you fail to hit the right calorie target. You must fuel yourself with sufficient energy to train hard and recover quickly. Here's how.

First, figure out how many calories it takes to maintain your current body weight with a sedentary lifestyle. Here's the formula: Body weight x 14 = estimated maintenance calories

EXAMPLE: A 190-pound man needs 2660 calories per day to remain at that weight. (190 x 14 = 2660)

Next, add or subtract 250 to 500 calories per day depending on whether you're in a shred phase or a mass phase.

MASS PHASE

Those who come to the program at less than 12 percent body fat will start with the done-for-you Mass meal plans included in part 10. You will be eating roughly 250 to 500 calories above your calculated maintenance weight, and your macronutrients will break down like this:

Mass Phase Training Days:
- Protein: 30 percent of your daily intake
- Carbohydrate: 50 percent of your daily intake
- Fat: 20 percent of your daily intake

Mass Phase Non-Training Days:
- Protein: 30 percent of your daily intake
- Carbohydrate: 20 percent of your daily intake
- Fat: 50 percent of your daily intake

As you can see, protein stays consistent on training and non-training days, as it's the building block for growth and repair. When you're training, your body needs carbs, which is why they are your dominant fuel source on training days. When you're not training, your body doesn't need as many carbs.

SHRED PHASE

Those who come to the program at above 12 percent body fat will start with the done-for-you Shred meal plans included in part 10.

You will be eating 250 to 500 calories below maintenance, and your macronutrients will break down like this:

Shred Phase Training Days:
- Protein: 30 percent of your daily intake
- Carbohydrate: 40 percent of your daily intake
- Fat: 30 percent of your daily intake

Shred Phase Non-Training Days:
- Protein: 50 percent of your daily intake
- Carbohydrate: 20 percent of your daily intake
- Fat: 30 percent of your daily intake

The logic is the same as the Mass meal plans when it comes to protein. Keep it high to promote muscle growth and prevent muscle loss. My rule of thumb is to always keep carbs higher on training days and lower on non-training days whether your goal is to gain muscle mass or shred fat.

These formulas are guidelines to begin. There is no "one-size-fits-all" perfect formula so pay close attention to how your body responds and adjust as needed.

Protein: The Body's Most Important Building Block

The word *protein* comes from the Greek *proteos*, meaning "the first one" or "the most important one." It's the body's most important building block. There are only twenty-one different amino acids from which all animal and plant proteins on earth are constructed. Nine of these twenty-one amino acids are known as *essential amino acids,* because the body is incapable of synthesizing them. They must come through food.

You need protein to help you pack on 30 pounds of muscle in the next 30 weeks. Protein is super awesome, but it's critical to understand that more is not better. Your daily protein requirement will stay consistent at 30 percent whether you are on the Mass or Shred meal plan.

Each meal should contain at least 20 to 30 grams of protein to hit the leucine threshold. Leucine is one of the three branched-chain amino acids (BCAAs) and is considered *the anabolic trigger*[45] because of its ability to stimulate skeletal muscle protein synthesis.

Avoid eating the same protein source twice in a day. Rotating protein sources is one of the best things you can do to optimize absorption and digestion, and it keeps your life more interesting. I've personally noticed better energy, less need for sleep, and faster recovery when I follow this rule. Here are two simple tips for protein rotation:

1) When you dine out, choose meats you rarely (or never) would prepare at home. This can be as simple as common steak, lamb, turkey, or pork chops, or meats you might never find in a regular grocery store. Try new sources to keep your diet exciting, such as alligator, buffalo, black bear, elk, kangaroo, ostrich, venison, wagyu, wild boar, and yak. If poultry is more your thing, try duck, goose, guinea fowl, pheasant, quail, and squab. You may not have heard of all of them, but somebody in your city probably has. Check ethnic markets, butcher shops, or search online.

2) Whey (milk protein) is not the only way to build muscle. Rotate milk protein powders (such as whey and casein) with plant protein powders (such as rice, pea, or hemp). My favorite protein powders can be found at the private customers link: getlivinglarge.com/musclebonuses.

Fat: The Key to Optimal Testosterone Production and Sex Drive

For many years, dietary fat got a bad rap. Viewed for decades as the evil ingredient that makes you sick, in truth, fat is essential to muscle building and health.

> *Viewed for decades as the evil ingredient that makes you sick, in truth, fat is essential to muscle building and health.*

Too little dietary fat will make your muscle building a living nightmare. The right amount of fat in your diet helps maintain optimal levels of testosterone,[46] which is responsible for muscle growth, strength, and sex drive.[47] This is why we keep fat at anywhere between 20 to 50 percent of your daily intake depending on the day and phase you're on.

I recommend you rotate seven key oils through your diet because they offer a wide variety of fatty acids and a broad spectrum of nutrients (so now you have zero excuses for being stuck on one oil): red palm oil, coconut oil, macadamia nut oil, extra virgin olive oil, hemp seed oil, walnut oil, and avocado oil. The oils to avoid because of their poor omega 6:3 ratio are safflower oil, peanut oil, sunflower oil, pumpkin seed oil, corn oil, pistachio oil, sesame oil, canola oil, and soybean oil.

Rotate foods so you get all three types of fat—saturated fats (butterfat from cows and goats, whole eggs, coconut oil, beef, cocoa butter, and chocolate), monounsaturated fats (oils, avocados, and most nuts), and polyunsaturated fats, which are also known as essential fatty acids because your body requires them for life. These are the omega-3 and omega-6 fatty acids (omega-3 fatty acids are most abundant in fish and fish oil supplements and omega-6 fatty acids are found in most vegetable oils and nuts).

One of my secrets to gaining muscle mass is rotating different nut butters into my protein shakes: almond butter, cashew butter, hazelnut butter, macadamia nut butter, pecan butter, walnut butter, and of course, everyone's favorite—peanut butter. Each has a variety of health benefits, and all are delicious.

Before you start slamming spoonful after spoonful, keep in mind that nut butters are just that: butters. Sure, it's good fat, but your body takes what it needs and turns the rest into stored fat. Always keep it pure—as few ingredients as possible. Ideally the ingredient list on your almond butter reads, "Almonds." Nothing else. Maybe, "Almonds, salt." But if reads something like, "Almonds, sugar, hydrogenated vegetable oil, salt, fancy molasses, mono and diglycerides," leave that jar on the shelf.

Carbs: You Need to Earn Them!

Carbohydrates are the only macronutrient we can live without, but not optimally. Carbs are like gasoline. They allow you to drive far and fast, meaning they allow you to train longer and harder. Carbs restock glycogen (80 percent of a workout is fueled by glycogen stores), prevent muscle breakdown, and keep life a lot tastier. A low glycogen state will compromise your ability to train hard. It's like taking a road trip with little gas in the tank.

But, "You need to deserve your carbs," says Charles Poliquin, one of the world's most accomplished strength coaches. If you're under 12 percent body fat, you can eat more carbs, and if you're over 12 percent body fat, you need to restrict them, but don't eliminate them, as outlined in the meal plans.

Regardless of body composition, reduce carb intake on non-training days. If your body doesn't have use for the immediate energy carbs provide, then it stocks the remainder in the liver and muscles through the process known as glycogenesis. When the liver and muscle reserves are full (approximately 500 grams or 2000 calories),[48] excess sugars get shuttled off to the adipose tissue to be stored as body fat.

Carbohydrates are usually divided into three types: complex, simple, and indigestible (fiber). This is based on their chemical structure and reflects how quickly they're digested and absorbed.

Complex carbohydrates are the staples that will get you jacked. They burn nice and slow and provide a long-lasting supply of energy. They are your go-to carb source for every meal except post-workout nutrition. This includes most fruits and vegetables, sweet potatoes, quinoa, oatmeal, brown rice, wild rice, and couscous.

Simple carbohydrates are fast acting and rapidly absorbed into the bloodstream. Consume these within the first 60 minutes after your workout to restock glycogen. My go-to whole food sources are carbs that are high on the glycemic index and low in fructose, so they are digested very quickly. This is when you can use a well-designed carb powder, as you'll learn in the supplement section. If you want

How to Use "Treat Meals" to Bulk Your Muscles, Not Your Belly

Back in the day, I used to put skinny guys on the "see food diet."

See food; eat it.

But after a while it started to backfire. Guys with great physique potential started ruining their bodies because they gained more fat than muscle. Now, my diet advice is based on science, strategy, and simplicity.

A lot of other experts recommend "cheat days" or "cheat meals" as a strategy to reward yourself and keep from going hog wild after a week or month of strict eating. I hate the term "cheat days" or "cheat meals." I call them "treat days" and "treat meals" because they are planned and they serve a positive muscle-building purpose.

Muscles grow on calories and even faster on nutrient-rich calories, so it's critical to hit your daily caloric intake; however, this poses a problem for guys who complain about having no appetite (if that's you, try taking in more B vitamins). Under-eating is a common reason guys can't manufacture new muscle tissue.

For skinny guys who are under 12 percent body fat and have trouble hitting their daily caloric target, my best advice is to swap out any one regular meal in the plan for a treat meal of similar macronutrients. For instance, post workout it's always carbs and protein, so instead of having chicken and potatoes, go for all-you-can-eat sushi. Let's say one of your meals is carbs, proteins, and fats, and you want to go to my favorite burger and fries spot, 5 Guys. Go for it. Or if you need a break from oatmeal and eggs in the morning, hit up your favorite pancake house for a big breakfast.

Use common sense and moderation. Don't subsist on pizza, burgers, and fries regularly. The goal is to make the rest of your meal plan easier to stick with. As long as you're under 12 percent body fat, your body will use those calories efficiently.

Some rules:

- It's a treat meal—NOT a treat day!
- When you stand up from the table, the meal is over.
- Never eat to the point of discomfort.
- Avoid alcohol with treat meals.
- Ideally, use on training days when you're hitting big body parts like back and legs.
- If your treat meals are hurting your physique more than helping, reevaluate the rules above.

Alcohol: You Booze, You Lose?

Alcohol is a fact of life, more so in some areas than others. Complete avoidance has a time and place, but it's not typically a sustainable solution for most people.

From an energy standpoint, alcohol contains 7 calories per gram,[56] so if you subtract the alcohol calories from your carb macros, you can consume alcohol in moderation without messing up your meal plan. The key is learning how many carbs are in your drink of choice.

I consider alcohol a "screwup" to muscle-building goals because it takes away from the body's ability to recover, restock glycogen, and optimize testosterone levels. However, I enjoy wine tastings with my wife and cracking open a new bottle of Scotch with my buddies, so I *plan* for these "screwups."

I've tried living by the "you do the booze, you lose" philosophy and it's only caused failure. Since I'm an extremist, if I have one drink I illogically think, "I've already screwed up, so I may as well finish the bottle." This often happens in a fancy setting, which leads to another bottle, dessert, and now it's game over. Here are some rules to guide your alcoholic decisions:

- Don't plan an epic workout the day after a party night. Alcohol lowers your testosterone levels for a couple of days.[57]
- Avoid alcohol if shredding fat is your top priority. Your body will use alcohol calories as fuel rather than fat stores and glycogen. This is because the metabolic by-product of alcohol, acetate, is toxic. So when you drink, fat burning stops until after you burn those calories off.[58]
- Do plan some interval cardio training to burn off the excess calories the next day, before they get stored as fat.
- Lower your fat intake and carb intake on the days you plan on drinking "hard."
- Plan your drinking for special occasions. I consider alcohol one of the finer delicacies in life, so I save my indulgences for wine tours, birthdays, holidays, anniversaries, and vacations.

Consistency: The "Best Diet" Is the One That You Follow

Everyone asks me, "What's the best juicer?"

I tell them, "The best juicer is the one that you use." It doesn't matter how many features or how much horsepower it has if it sits idle on a shelf.

Same holds true with your meal plans.

Just because a plan looks good on paper, if you can't follow it, you'll fail to achieve your goals. Don't waste time trying to find the "best" diet. The best diet is the one that you *follow*. You can build muscle on a lot of different meal plans if you follow the right principles and adjust the plan to how you're responding (or not responding).

The best diet is the one that you follow.

Never underestimate the small dietary choices you must make each day, because they add up. Each situation presents an opportunity to make a decision that will either help your goals or hurt your goals. If you make enough "help" decisions, the accumulation of those will speed you toward your goal.

To gain 30 pounds of muscle in 30 weeks, you'll make a lot of choices that might not seem appealing in the moment. You can't have treat meals every meal. You'll have to interrupt what you're doing to grab one of your meals on time. You'll need to say no to alcohol on more occasions than you'll partake. You'll need to pay attention to your portion sizes instead of mindlessly eating. You'll need to eat when sometimes you don't feel like it.

At the end of the day, no diet works for you. You work the diet. If it were easy, everyone would have bulging muscles and six-pack abs. It comes down to personal accountability for the choices you make and making more help decisions than hurt decisions.

The Devil Is in the Dose, Never in the Food Itself

I got an email with the headline, "Which vegetable makes you fat?"

Shaking my head, I opened it and saw three choices: "Click here if you think it's spinach, here if you think it's kale, here if you think it's broccoli."

"Are you kidding me?" I muttered. "I've never met a single person in my life who's gotten fat on any vegetable!"

Many marketers try to get your attention with sensationalism and fearmongering. If you see a headline that reads, "NEVER eat these foods," take it as suspicious because many of these marketers have good intentions, but they fail to reveal the truth: The devil is in the dose.

Every food that gets labeled "good" can also have an unhealthy or "bad" dose, just as every food that is labeled "bad" can have a perfectly acceptable dose that will do no harm to either your health or your physique goals. And I mean *any* food—even if it's trans fat, sugar, artificial sweeteners, genetically modified anything, high fructose corn syrup, nonlocal foods, refined white flour, or that "toxic" chemical you can't pronounce. Forget the hype. As long as you don't overdo it with any single item, there's no such thing as a "bad food."

The devil is always in the dose, not the food itself.

A teaspoon of sugar in your coffee can make it the highlight of your day. Pounding pounds of sugar in the form of sweets, sodas, snacks, dressings, and baked goods will give you diabetes.

Follow these simple and practical rules:

1) **Cook at home as much as possible.** When you dine out, you can't control how fresh the ingredients are, what goes into your food, or how they cook it. Usually restaurants use more fat than you would use at home.

2) **Avoid foods that make you feel like hell.** Obviously, if you're violently allergic to a food, you shouldn't ever eat it. If you eat something and feel like crap, you might have a mild food allergy or intolerance. Visit a naturopathic doctor to help you find out what you're sensitive to and avoid those foods.

3) **The best foods are the ones you can find in nature.** Eighty percent of your nutrition should come from unprocessed whole foods. Another 10 percent should come from minimally processed foods, such as canned tuna, tomato sauce, or salad dressing with chemical-free ingredients (example: olive oil, garlic, vinegar, salt, pepper). And you can have up to 10 percent of your diet from the heavily processed category (packaged foods with ingredients listed that sound more like a recipe for a chemistry class experiment than anything you could make at home). Likely, this is where your treat meals would fit in. At the grocery store, shop the perimeter where the fresh foods are stocked. The middle aisles typically are laden with heavily processed foods, so avoid them, or go in to find something specific.

Arm Yourself with the Only Kitchen Tools You Need

I used to be terrified of cooking. It seemed like an extreme sport. I thought I'd need tons of special equipment. But after hiring a professional chef for hours of cooking lessons, I learned the truth. The list of essential kitchen tools is short.

Here are the essentials that, when combined with a little know-how, can get you making tasty meals in no time: a cutting board, a chef's knife, a vegetable peeler, a can opener, a paring knife, and a good set of steak knives. If you want to make a big investment upfront for a set of knives that will last, go for a full-blown set of professional knives or a top home brand like Cutco. (Did you know I paid my way through university selling Cutco knives on the side? True story!)

Other essential equipment: a good spatula for stir-fries and omelets, mixing bowls, a large and a small saucepot, and a nontoxic frying pan. Get a set of stainless steel measuring spoons, and grab a spice rack. They are incredibly cheap, and you'll be able to make flavorful meals. Buy a meat thermometer, so you don't overcook your meat until it tastes like a dried old towel.

If you can afford it, pick up a quality blender. I bought a Vitamix ten years ago for $400, and it's the best money I've ever spent. You can make your own homemade shakes and even nut butters. The first blender I ever bought was a vertical handheld blender for $40 and I must have made hundreds of shakes with it.

To optimize your health, buy a juicer and start your day with a few of your favorite greens blended up to infuse your body with a ton of vitamins and minerals. I do.

A slow cooker and a George Foreman grill is a must for busy people on the go. You can cook a few days' worth of food with these bad boys.

Last, but very important, stock your kitchen with big eating tools—big plates, big cups, big forks—big everything. To get big you need to eat big, so it only makes sense to have big eating equipment to support your goal.

Invest in Cooking Lessons and Cook Like a Pro

I met a bodybuilder who was 230 pounds and 5 percent body fat. I asked him, "How the heck do you maintain your physique?"

"It's easy, man."

"What do you mean, 'It's easy?' I've never heard anyone say that!"

"My wife knows how to cook. Her chicken breast is amazing. It's never raw. It's moist. It's juicy."

That got my attention. As a young guy, I didn't get the importance of having a few good cooking skills and the difference it could make.

After I got married, my wife and I were very, very busy. We were working from home, and we both went to extremes with our diet preparing for photo shoots. We realized our main limitation was that we didn't know how to make our food taste good.

We enrolled in cooking lessons with Chef Amy Stoddart in Toronto, Ontario, and just learning a few tricks made a huge difference. First, I learned how to create simple seasonings and marinades. I learned time-saving tips to prepare my meals in advance; how to make meals in as little as five minutes; how to use residual heat to never overcook my meat; how to chop like a pro; and how to produce restaurant-quality meals inside my own home.

To get you started, I'm giving you my simple no-nonsense meal plans to follow. When those start getting bland and boring, I have a resource called *Max Muscle Recipe Guide & Gourmet Meal Plans* that comes as a bonus with my Living Large Inner Circle membership site, where you can get more than forty cooking lessons with my wife, Chef Amy, and me. We will teach you more than fifty gourmet recipes, so you can substitute more tasty meals for the meals that may be getting bland. You can learn more at getlivinglarge.com/musclebonuses.

PART 10

The Done-for-You Mass and Shred Meal Plans

The nutrition part is vital. You're in the gym one hour a day. The other 23 hours, you'll make or break your success by what you put into your body. To make this easy, here is a complete set of done-for-you meal plans. They are nutritionally balanced, wholesome, and designed to help you recover so you can build your body bigger and stronger than ever before. (They are not gourmet. If you want gourmet options, go to getlivinglarge.com/musclebonuses and find out how you can get access to gourmet recipes that are designed by a professional chef.)

I've given you meals for both phases of bodybuilding—Mass (for building muscle) and Shred (to cut the fat and reveal your ripped body). These are the optimal plans to help you lose fat and build muscle. You'll also find two sets of meal plans—one to follow on training days, the other to use on non-training days.

Tailor the meal plans to fit your individual goals. If you're over 12 percent body fat, start with the Shred phase, and if you're under 12 percent, begin with Mass phase. Choose one to start.

Next, figure out your optimal caloric intake (see page 190). Whatever your calculation says, round the number down or up to the nearest increment. For example, if you get 2,750 calories as your target intake, and you're in a Shred phase, go down to 2,500 calories. If you are in a Mass phase, round up to the 3,000-calorie plan. Re-assess your body weight every three weeks to determine when you should transition to a new meal plan. It is critical that you are following the meal plans at least 90 percent of the time to ensure that the changes to your nutrition help you and don't hurt you.

The two main excuses I hear from guys regarding nutrition are "I don't know how to cook," and "I don't have time to cook." These simple, no-nonsense meal plans are easy to make and don't take a lot of time to prepare. So no excuses!

[CONTINUED]

MEAL/FOOD	CALORIES	CARBS (G)	PROTEIN (G)	FATS (G)
MEAL 6				
1 scoop whey protein	105	0	25	1
1 cup cherry juice	135	35	2	0
1 tbsp coconut oil	117	0	0	14
Totals:	**357**	**35**	**27**	**15**
DAILY TOTALS	**3,517**	**190**	**271**	**199**

4,000-Calorie Meal Plan – 20/30/50 (Carbs/Protein/Fats)

MEAL/FOOD	CALORIES	CARBS (G)	PROTEIN (G)	FATS (G)
MEAL 1				
6 oz lean meat	287	0	53	6
1 tbsp olive oil	119	0	0	14
¼ cup raw nuts	206	7	8	18
2 tbsp nut butter	188	6	8	16
Totals:	**800**	**13**	**69**	**54**
MEAL 2				
1 scoop whey protein	105	0	25	1
¼ cup raw nuts	206	7	8	18
½ avocado	161	9	2	15
Totals:	**472**	**16**	**35**	**34**
MEAL 3				
6 oz lean meat	287	0	53	6
1 tbsp olive oil	119	0	0	14
1 cup brown rice	216	45	5	2
1 cup vegetables	23	4	2	0
5 oz olives	236	10	0	19
Totals:	**881**	**59**	**60**	**41**
MEAL 4				
6 oz lean meat	287	0	53	6
1 tbsp olive oil	119	0	0	14
1 cup vegetables	23	4	2	0
½ avocado	161	9	2	15
Totals:	**590**	**13**	**57**	**35**

MEAL/FOOD	CALORIES	CARBS (G)	PROTEIN (G)	FATS (G)
MEAL 5				
5 whole eggs	388	3	32	27
30g light Havarti cheese	118	1	8	9
¼ cup raw nuts	206	7	8	18
2 slices 12-grain toast	220	42	10	3
Totals:	**932**	**53**	**58**	**57**
MEAL 6				
1 scoop whey protein	105	0	25	1
1 cup cherry juice	135	35	2	0
1 tbsp coconut oil	117	0	0	14
Totals:	**357**	**35**	**27**	**15**
DAILY TOTALS	**4,032**	**189**	**306**	**236**

4,500-Calorie Meal Plan – 20/30/50 (Carbs/Protein/Fats)

MEAL/FOOD	CALORIES	CARBS (G)	PROTEIN (G)	FATS (G)
MEAL 1				
6 oz lean meat	287	0	53	6
1 tbsp olive oil	119	0	0	14
¼ cup raw nuts	206	7	8	18
2 tbsp nut butter	188	6	8	16
Totals:	**800**	**13**	**69**	**54**
MEAL 2				
1 scoop whey protein	105	0	25	1
¼ cup raw nuts	206	7	8	18
½ avocado	161	9	2	15
1 medium banana	105	27	0	1
Totals:	**577**	**43**	**35**	**35**
MEAL 3				
6 oz lean meat	287	0	53	6
1 tbsp olive oil	119	0	0	14
2 cups brown rice	432	90	10	4
1 cup vegetables	23	4	2	0
1 cup berries	46	11	1	0
5 oz olives	236	10	0	19
Totals:	**1,143**	**115**	**66**	**43**

CONTINUED

TRAINING DAY: SHRED PHASE MEAL PLANS

1,500-Calorie Meal Plan – 40/30/30 (Carbs/Protein/Fats)

MEAL/FOOD	CALORIES	CARBS (G)	PROTEIN (G)	FATS (G)
MEAL 1				
2 oz lean meat	94	0	18	2
½ cup raw nuts	413	14	15	36
2 tbsp nut butter	94	3	4	8
Totals:	**601**	**17**	**37**	**46**
1-3 HOURS PRE-WORKOUT				
1 cup quinoa	222	39	8	4
2 cups vegetables	46	8	4	0
Totals:	**268**	**47**	**12**	**4**
INTRA-WORKOUT				
20g carb powder	75	20	0	0
10g whey isolate	34	0	8	0
Totals:	**109**	**20**	**8**	**0**
15 TO 60 MINUTES POST-WORKOUT				
40g carb powder	150	40	0	0
25g whey isolate	86	0	21	0
Totals:	**236**	**40**	**21**	**0**
MEAL 2				
2 oz lean meat	94	0	18	2
½ cup quinoa	111	20	4	2
Totals:	**205**	**20**	**22**	**4**
MEAL 3				
½ cup fat-free cottage cheese	40	3	7	0
1 cup vegetables	23	4	2	0
Totals:	**63**	**7**	**9**	**0**
DAILY TOTALS	**1,482**	**151**	**109**	**54**

2,000-Calorie Meal Plan – 40/30/30 (Carbs/Protein/Fats)

MEAL/FOOD	CALORIES	CARBS (G)	PROTEIN (G)	FATS (G)
MEAL 1				
3 oz lean meat	140	0	26	3
½ cup raw nuts	413	14	15	36
Totals:	**553**	**14**	**41**	**39**
1-3 HOURS PRE-WORKOUT				
3 oz lean meat	140	0	26	3
1 cup quinoa	222	39	8	4
1 cup vegetables	23	4	2	0
Totals:	**385**	**43**	**36**	**7**
INTRA-WORKOUT				
45g carb powder	169	45	0	0
15g whey isolate	52	0	12	0
Totals:	**221**	**45**	**12**	**0**
15 TO 60 MINUTES POST-WORKOUT				
50g carb powder	188	50	0	0
40g whey isolate	138	0	33	0
Totals:	**326**	**50**	**33**	**0**
MEAL 2				
3 oz lean meat	140	0	26	3
1 tbsp olive oil	119	0	0	14
½ cup quinoa	111	20	4	2
1 medium orange	62	15	1	0
Totals:	**432**	**35**	**31**	**19**
MEAL 3				
1 cup fat-free cottage cheese	80	6	14	0
2 cups vegetables	46	8	4	0
Totals:	**126**	**14**	**18**	**0**
DAILY TOTALS	**2,043**	**201**	**171**	**65**

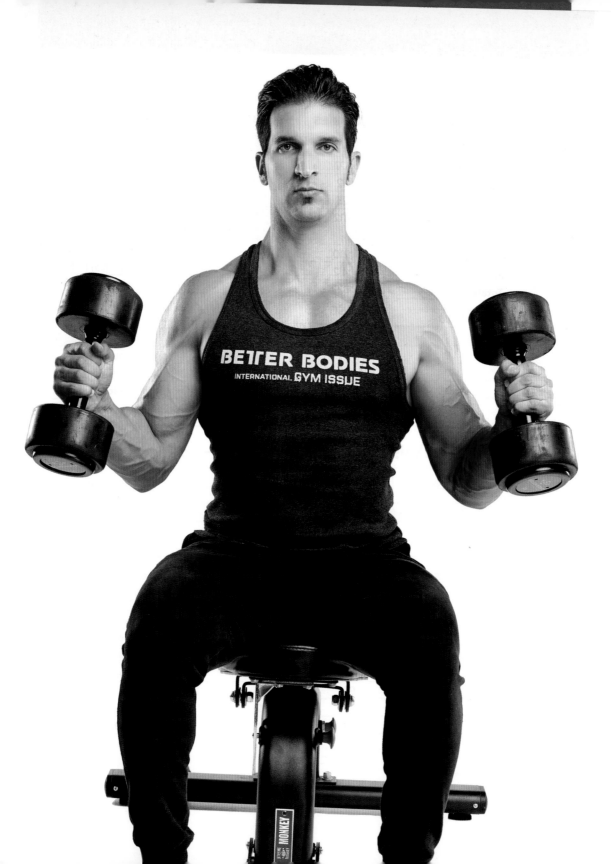

2,000-Calorie Meal Plan – 40/30/30 (Carbs/Protein/Fats)

MEAL/FOOD	CALORIES	CARBS (G)	PROTEIN (G)	FATS (G)
MEAL 1				
3 oz lean meat	140	0	26	3
½ cup raw nuts	413	14	15	36
Totals:	**553**	**14**	**41**	**39**
1–3 HOURS PRE-WORKOUT				
3 oz lean meat	140	0	26	3
1 cup quinoa	222	39	8	4
1 cup vegetables	23	4	2	0
Totals:	**385**	**43**	**36**	**7**
INTRA-WORKOUT				
45g carb powder	169	45	0	0
15g whey isolate	52	0	12	0
Totals:	**221**	**45**	**12**	**0**
15 TO 60 MINUTES POST-WORKOUT				
50g carb powder	188	50	0	0
40g whey isolate	138	0	33	0
Totals:	**326**	**50**	**33**	**0**
MEAL 2				
3 oz lean meat	140	0	26	3
1 tbsp olive oil	119	0	0	14
½ cup quinoa	111	20	4	2
1 medium orange	62	15	1	0
Totals:	**432**	**35**	**31**	**19**
MEAL 3				
1 cup fat-free cottage cheese	80	6	14	0
2 cups vegetables	46	8	4	0
Totals:	**126**	**14**	**18**	**0**
DAILY TOTALS	**2,043**	**201**	**171**	**65**

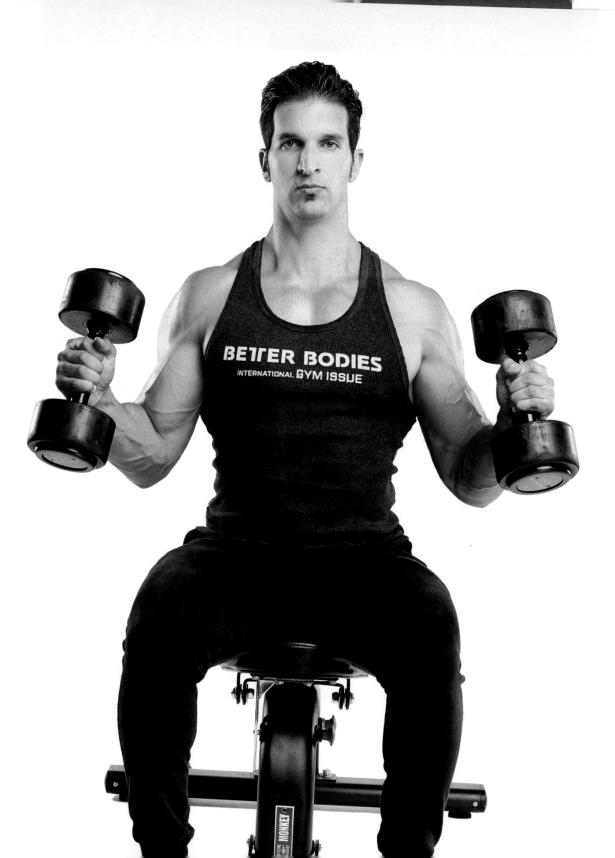

PART 11

Supplements That Actually Work (Don't Worry, This Part Is Short)

Finding good information on supplements can be a daunting task. It seems everywhere you look, you find conflicting claims on the good, the bad, and the garbage. One day you feel like you should be taking everything, and the next you're sure that all of it is worthless.

Sorting out the truth becomes simpler as soon as you understand that supplements don't actually have "druglike" properties, as the ads suggest, nor are they adequate replacements for healthy meals. Supplements are exactly what the name states: "supplements" to a good diet. As basic as this sounds, it's this realization that has allowed me to experiment with supplements without losing my mind or burning a hole in my wallet.

I like to separate supplements into two categories: the workers and the situational supplements.

The Workers

Workers are the supplements to take all year round, no matter what. For me, this includes vitamins, minerals, fish oils, probiotics, and enzymes. If you're deficient in the "workers," then your body will lack the staples to maintain optimal health. Investing in these types of supplements is the best use of your supplement budget. You should always put your money toward the "worker" supplements before you spend anything on the next category.

Situational Supplements

For most of you, the whole conversation around situational supplements is premature. But suffice to say that situational supplements can be useful when you are preparing for a specific athletic event, photo shoot, or competition.

Full Disclosure

In this section I will provide a link where you'll find my exact product recommendations. And, yes, I earn a commission if you purchase any of the products through the links I provide. I disclose this because some people may decide to discredit my recommendations because of that, which is silly, because, guess what? I could promote any supplement in the world and still earn a commission! Every single supplement company in the world cuts commission checks to their affiliates and partners! Still, I only promote the products that I've extensively used on myself and have recommended to my family, friends, and clients.

I've been promoting the same brands and products for a long time, but as you know, nothing stays the same forever. That's why I opted to put my recommendations on a live webpage, rather than here in the print book. That way, I can add new excellent products that may come along, and if a supplement company changes ownership and/or loses quality, I can remove them and all their products from my page.

No matter what I recommend here or what you choose to purchase, never let supplements distract you from the main essentials—eating right and training hard.

Do You Earn the Right to Take Supplements?

The gym I train at is full of young guys who often approach me for supplement advice. "Vince, what's the best pre-workout supplement?" "What kind of creatine should I take?" or "What's your favorite mass gainer?" "Do you think I should get this fat burner?" "Can you recommend a good testosterone booster?"

I can answer all of these questions, but I don't—unless they can answer my questions: "How many calories are you consuming daily? What are your macros? How is your body responding?"

If people can't tell me their calories and macros, or provide clear feedback about their progress, I don't give them an answer. Not because I'm a jerk, but because their priorities are mixed up. They are shopping for supplements before they've even seen what they can accomplish with whole food.

That goes for you, too. Don't ask me any of these questions unless you are consistently (at least 80 percent of the time) hitting your target calories and macros. If you aren't, then put down the supplement catalogs, review the meal plans in this book, and go to the grocery store.

If this sounds harsh, too bad. It's annoying to hear these guys fixate on supplements that may have a 10 percent impact when they are neglecting the 90 percent that will transform their physiques.

I'm just as guilty as the next guy who wishes supplements were magical! But there is absolutely no substitute for consistently hitting your calorie and macro targets. If you're not compliant with your meal plan at least 80 percent of the time, you can forget about any degree of muscular development, because supplements can't correct a bad diet, regardless of which ones you take. Over the years, I've become a bigger and bigger believer in nutritional supplements to bio-optimize the body, fix deficiencies, and increase performance, but don't assume that they should, or even could, take the place of a well-designed, healthy, and balanced nutritional plan. The only supplements I used when I gained over 40 pounds of lean mass were whey protein, creatine, vitamins and minerals, and some fish oils.

> ### *There is absolutely no substitute for consistently hitting your calorie and macro targets.*

Still, I doubt you'll come close to realizing your full muscle-growth potential without the addition of a few well-chosen, high quality nutritional supplements. In this book, I'm only going to focus on four.

The first two supplements I recommend in the following sections are "workers" (as discussed earlier), and the second two are "fuel." The "workers" aid your body's ability to absorb and utilize the nutrients that the "fuel" can provide. Nutrients can't work as well for you if you're not fully absorbing them.

One caveat that applies to all: get a full physical exam before taking any supplement and consult with your doctor. However, most traditionally trained physicians don't know jack about nutrition or supplements, so you may want to seek out a naturopathic doctor or a very smart and up-to-date nutritionist. My naturopathic doctor reads my blood work and tells me exactly which supplements I'm wasting my money on and points out beneficial supplements I've never even heard of to make up for my body's deficiencies. Do your own research before making a decision on what to take. For more information on naturopathic doctors I recommend, go to getlivinglarge.com/musclebonuses.

How to Build More Muscle with Less Protein

Everybody has been brainwashed that pounding more protein equals more muscle. However, your first goal must be to optimize the protein you're already consuming.

Without getting too complicated, enzymes are key to your body's life force. Enzymes are the sparks that make everything happen, and without them you cannot possibly maximize muscular growth. Enzymes help digest your food, break down proteins into amino acids, stimulate your brain, provide cellular energy, and help repair all the cells, tissues, and organs of your body.

Nature designed food to break itself down in the digestive tract. However, modern man has gone against nature's ways. As soon as you heat any food to 118 degrees Fahrenheit, it kills all the enzymes that exist in whole foods.[59] That and the processed foods, irradiated foods, foods sprayed with pesticides, chemical fertilizers, or grown in mineral deficient soils is why an average forty-year-old has 40 percent less enzyme reserves than a child.[60]

Dr. Howell's book *Enzyme Nutrition* points to evidence suggesting enzyme-deficient diets are a potential contributing factor in disease. Dr. Howell also states that by age twenty-seven, for individuals who train intensely, most of the protease functioning in the body has shut down as the body recognizes it cannot keep up to the metabolic pace. If you examine the careers of most superstar athletes, their performance tends to peak around age twenty-six to twenty-eight and then starts to decline.[61]

One of the biggest insider secrets I learned from the director of education for BiOptimizers, advisor for the American Anti-Cancer Institute, and three-time All Natural Bodybuilding Champion Wade Lightheart is that the key to bigger and faster muscle gains is extreme amino acid absorption. This is how steroids work, but of course, steroids eventually cause you to crash and burn. So how can we do this naturally?

A potent proteolytic enzyme formulation.

Proteolytic enzymes replenish your enzyme pools so that you can become more efficient at absorbing protein and get more benefit from what you eat, making it easier to gain muscle long-term.

Taking a potent proteolytic enzyme formula can keep you from building up undigested protein that can lead to a multitude of degenerative diseases. And there are other health benefits. To learn more about how to increase your muscle gains without increasing your protein intake, go to getlivinglarge.com/musclebonuses.

The War in Your Gut: Are You Losing?

Over the course of your lifetime, approximately one hundred tons of food will pass through your digestive system, and the digestive tract is host to more than four hundred different types of bacteria that outnumber *all* the cells in your body. Here's the breakdown:

- 10 percent are good ("friendly" bacteria)
- 10 percent are bad ("unfriendly" bacteria)
- 80 percent are opportunists—meaning they will proliferate, depending on environmental circumstances.

As long as you have plenty of friendly bacteria, the unfriendly bacteria will be kept under control. However, changes in environment, diet, stress levels, toxic load, hydration, enzyme content of food, and especially the use of antibiotics can upset this delicate balance.

Left unchecked, the "bad" bacteria in your gut tends to get stronger as you age, especially if you've ever taken antibiotics (one of the side effects is extremely hardy bad bacteria that survived a full-on antibiotic attack). Antibiotics destroy both good and bad bacteria, so if you've ever taken antibiotics in your life, you've most likely compromised this important balance of bacteria in your gut, weakening your body's ability to function—and build muscle.

"Good" bacteria assists in assimilating the nutrients you take in, but there's not a lot of it, and it's under constant threat. Consumption of aspartame, genetically modified organisms (GMOs),[62] chemicals, and environmental toxins all cause mutations in gut bacteria,[63] reducing your ability to absorb your food.[64] Also, changes in diet and psychological stress can affect gut bacteria and its ability to work for you.

You want the protein you consume to help make more muscle, adding size and strength to transform that skinny guy frame. But most guys are only seeing a fraction of the muscle-building results they should because there's a secret war being waged in the intestines about where that protein should end up, and right now, most guys (probably you) are losing.

A regular probiotic supplement is not enough to shift the balance. And that stuff they put in yogurt and sell you through the grocery store is useless. Manufacturers add so many junk food ingredients along with it that they counteract all the good that the probiotics would deliver.[65]

For info on the best available today, go to getlivinglarge.com/musclebonuses.

Protein Powders: Whey Is Not the Only Way

No matter how many people ask me, I still get the same three questions on protein powders, so let's address each one.

1) **Is protein powder necessary?** Solid food is always better than processed protein powders. Yet modern life does not always allow us to consume our daily caloric target in solid food form each day. Protein powders can help. The fastest way to reach your muscle-building goals is to reserve shakes for peri-workout nutrition, and no more than one homemade shake per day. Don't make the mistake believing that protein powders can take the place of solid food. You'll end up staying soft and scrawny.

Live by this mantra: To look solid, eat solid food.

2) **Does protein powder really work?** Studies have shown that protein supplements, such as protein powder, can increase muscle mass and improve exercise performance, particularly when taken shortly after training sessions.[66] They work best when you respect their role as supplements and avoid using them as a fallback for laziness and a lack of preparation.

3) **What is the best protein powder?** There is no such thing. Each one has pros and cons depending on your goal.

Just like you should consume a variety of whole food protein sources, rotate your protein powders too. For instance, casein is great for cooking. You can make some awesome cheesecake, ice cream, and muffins due to its gel-forming properties. For muscle building, it's a waste of money. Soy is as good as other protein sources in terms of amino acids and protein quality; however, it can be a hormonal disaster, which is why I avoid it.[67,68] Rice and pea protein are bundled together because they are both incomplete protein sources, but by mixing them, you have a complete vegan source. It's a great option for people allergic to eggs, dairy, and soy. Egg protein is good for variety but there is no evidence to support its usage over other protein powders.[69]

Here are my top two options:

Whey. Whey protein makes up 20 percent of total milk protein. Whey is acknowledged for its superior amino acid profile, high cysteine content, fast digestion, and mixture of peptides. However, its practical benefits are far overstated in marketing copy. Sure, it digests faster. But the speed of digestion does not make a big difference to your body, so don't get all excited about "fast absorption." Personally, I think the whole absorption-rate debate is blown out of proportion. I've tried them all, and I've noticed zero difference. Just focus on getting your daily protein intake and use a high-quality protein powder that you can afford.

Also, don't worry if you're using a whey concentrate, isolate, or hydrolysate. Frankly, you can use whey protein any time of the day. I reserve it for peri-workout.

Hemp. Hemp protein is one of the few plant proteins that contain all twenty-one amino acids used by humans, including the nine essential amino acids that must come from diet.[70] Hemp also contains a perfect ratio of essential fatty acids along with massive quantities of insoluble fiber, which is essential for digestive health.[71] Hemp boosts testosterone levels with the most potent source of essential fatty acids in nature, increases protein synthesis naturally because of its high globulin protein,[72] boosts your body's "friendly" bacteria,[73] switches your body from an acidic state to an alkaline state, and helps eliminate intestinal toxemia (that bloated belly look).

To view my recommendations for protein powders, go to getlivinglarge.com/musclebonuses.

Carbohydrate Powder:
The Ultimate Muscle-Building Solution

With so many new carb powders hitting the market, sorting them all out has become as confusing as protein powders. Carb powders "spike" your insulin and help restock glycogen before your next workout, prevent muscle breakdown, maximize performance, and help you meet your high carbohydrate needs.

I have experimented with virtually every carb powder on the market: Gatorade, dextrose, maltodextrin, Karbo-Lyn, Vitargo, highly branched cyclic dextrins (HBCD) and SuperStarch. Don't lose sleep over which one "absorbs faster." Not a big deal.

I recommend you try a few and pay attention to gut issues. If you experience bloating, diarrhea, or gastrointestinal discomfort, switch it up and try a different one.

During your workout you can substitute carb powder with any sports drink, red berry juice, or pineapple juice. After your workout you can substitute carb powder with rice cakes, white rice, cornflakes, maple syrup, or honey. To view my recommended carb powders, go to getlivinglarge.com/musclebonuses.

PART 12

A No-Nonsense Guide to Living Large Outside of the Gym

Let's first be clear. To me, living large has nothing to do with the Urban Dictionary's definition, which is *"Living with an extravagant or self-indulgent lifestyle."*

To me, living large is not about the size of your wallet, or even your biceps. It's about how you show up. When you're truly living large, you'll be an action-taker, dedicated to serving others. You'll get outside of your comfort zone, betting on yourself, and inspiring others while you demonstrate a spirit of gratitude and humility.

> *When you're truly living large, you'll be moved to a place of gratitude and humility as you realize all experiences, even difficult ones, turn out to be unexpected gifts.*

Build Muscle to Serve, Not to Be Served

Muscle is very hard to build and calorically expensive to maintain. One key question to ask yourself about building muscle is, Why do you want it?

The true motivation has nothing to do with muscle itself. Virtually every guy gets into muscle building to mask an insecurity. They want an ego boost. They hope the muscle will fill a void in their life. They want an identity that includes confidence, respect, money, power, and sex. And muscle *can* give you all of that.

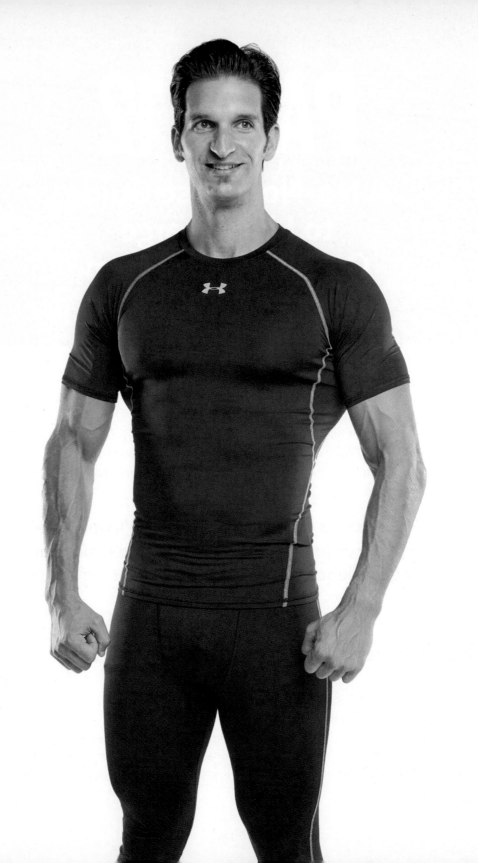

The problem comes when you try to use muscle like an armor to hide a gaping void inside. You will never be able to fill an internal void by building a better body. And if you try, be prepared to get a complex. No matter how much muscle you build, you'll end up feeling unfulfilled, empty, and probably lonely.

When I finally dropped my "Skinny Vinny" label for good, I quickly realized that becoming obsessed with chasing more self-serving muscle for the sake of getting *bigger* would lead to a dead end.

> ### *You will never be able to fill an internal void by building a better body.*

If gaining 41 pounds of scale weight without adding any fat to my midsection couldn't make me happy, how would another 10 to 20 pounds be any better? I saw early on that it would lead to a self-absorbed and selfish lifestyle that was all about me, me, me, and leave no room for anyone to get close.

This reality inspired me to find a way to use my efforts in the gym to go beyond my own self-interests and serve others. This is one of the reasons I stayed in the fitness industry as a personal trainer. It's one of the reasons I started my online fitness business. And it's one of the reasons I started doing live events and running Muscle Camps, which you can watch on my YouTube channel. It is one of the reasons I wrote this book.

By sharing the same knowledge that helped me transform, I have a bigger purpose than my own selfish gains. I have created a world where others count on me to be there for them and to give them hope.

> ### *Living large is about staying humble and inspiring others. Living large is being a walking billboard of "trading up" in life.*

Living large is about staying humble and inspiring others. Living large is being a walking billboard of "trading up" in life. Living large is not bragging about how far you've come or viewing anyone with a lesser body as a lesser person. Living large is about remembering where you started and helping others get to where you are with the hope that they pay it forward, too. Even on the smallest level, every time you're in the gym, you have the opportunity to live large by encouraging a new member, or giving someone with poor technique some help, or complimenting someone on their progress.

Take Massive Action (Don't Just Think or Talk About It)

Back in 2005, I was invited into a one-on-one Internet marketing coaching program where the price to play was $7,500 for a six-month course to learn how to create digital information products, so that

I could create a second stream of income and profit from my knowledge. It was a huge investment for me at the time. I had to shuffle money around and use more than one credit card to cover it. But I signed up and sprung into action despite the risk of failure and being outside of my comfort zone.

Within six months, I'd created my first e-book, *No-Nonsense Muscle Building: Skinny Guy Secrets to Insane Muscle Gain*; put up a website, www.vincedelmontefitness.com; and started making sales. In my first year online, I made exactly $10,000. In my second year, I made $101,000—more than at my job as a personal trainer, so I decided to fire my boss. In my third year, I made $350,000. In my fourth year, I made $850,000. Before the age of thirty, I made my first million dollars and was well on my way to the lifestyle of my dreams.

I'm not the biggest, strongest, or leanest guy. I'm not the smartest guy. But it's rarely the smartest person who wins. It's the one who takes massive action and is willing to work. That whole time, I worked 40 hours a week at my job, and 40 hours a week online. I didn't take any days off. No one could stop me.

Some may find these numbers big, some will see them as small. Income numbers don't define me, just like the size of my biceps doesn't define me. What matters is that I got results not by thinking about it, not by talking about it, but by taking action. The cool thing about taking action is that things start to happen. Sales pages go live. Products are born. Your first affiliate promotes. Customers rave. Money flows. You start to hire. Systems emerge. Your brand gains popularity. Recognition fuels the fire. You went from a skeptic to a believer, and now you're inspiring others to follow your path. It seems magical, but it's not. It's because you took action. Persistent action. Focused action. Massive action.

There are no shortcuts to anywhere worth going.

There are no shortcuts to anywhere worth going. It starts with a decision you make on one single day, and taking action that compounds until you are living your dreams.

Avoid Broken Focus

Focus is saying "yes" to one thing and defending that "yes" by saying a thousand "nos."[74]

People often don't understand the power of focus because they are unable to say "no" to nonessential activities. But focus has rewards. And broken focus has consequences.

Back in high school, I was on the track team, and I was thinking of joining some of my friends on the soccer team in the fall. Most of my friends did every sport—basketball, soccer, track—and I thought maybe this was a time I should be trying out lots of things.

My track coach took me aside and pointed out the top runners in the country, saying, "Want to race against this guy? You think this guy plays soccer on the side?"

I realized then that, if I wanted greater rewards, I had to focus—focus on one thing and sacrifice the others. I loved soccer. I actually liked playing soccer more than running, but I saw more of a future with my running, so I focused.

The result: I made the university track team. I got to travel all over Canada and the United States for meets. Very few of my friends took a sport beyond high school. But I got more out of my sports experience because I was willing to commit to a single focus and sacrifice other sports.

Focus has rewards.
And broken focus has consequences.

The same could be said about business. I love the saying, "Go an inch wide and a mile deep." That's what I've done with the skinny guy market. I've gone deep. I've built my online fitness business around helping men to gain their first 30 pounds of muscle, then their next 20 pounds of muscle, and finally another 10 pounds of muscle. I'm not trying to be the fat-loss guy, or the strength guy, or the "insert next flashy trend" guy. I'm focused on skinny guys. In business, this idea sounds counterintuitive because it seems like you're shrinking your market, but by going deeper and not wider, it in fact creates more success.

The same could be said about women in your life. You can choose to experience lots of women in a shallow way, or focus on one woman and go deep. You will never experience the rewards of focusing on one woman if you're always playing the field.

And it's the same with training. I have shown you three 10-week phases. Each phase and each workout has a primary focus. To get the best results, focus on one goal at a time and go as deep with it as you can.

Get Blood in the Game

Every time I sign up for a fitness model competition, I've got to get some blood in the game. It helps me do my best. You might say it's motivating enough just to know I have to go up on stage and parade around in a skimpy bikini and pose for a bunch of strangers while being judged against other guys who are absolutely shredded and ripped too. But having just my ego on the line isn't what does it for me. I'm not looking to take the top prize on stage, anyway. I'm happy to finish in the top ten. I know I don't have the best physique, and I'm not prepared to do what it takes to have it.

I am more interested in leveraging the experience to grow my online fitness business, and that means I've got even more at stake—my livelihood, my reputation, my wife, my family, my finances, and my credibility.

When I decide to compete, the first thing I do is announce it on social media. I tell my entire audience to follow along with me. I hire a top expert coach. I also leverage the experience, and often tie it to a new information product, as I did with *Stage Shredded Status*. So, if I have four weeks until the contest, and it seems like my body's not changing, I'm going to say to myself, "I have to keep going. The stakes are so high."

ACKNOWLEDGMENTS

It's amazing this book is finally here. There was a point where I thought it would remain an idea. Six years ago, my good friend Joel Marion helped me write a book proposal for what was going to be called "The Skinny Guy Savior," but for some reason I never got pen to paper to write the darn book, so it sat on the backlog for years.

So, here are the people I wish to thank who helped trigger a series of events that finally put this book into your hands.

First of all, to my parents, Luciano and Rosetta. It's amazing to say that my parents are my best friends. Thank you for inspiring me to read at an early age and letting me read everything from fantasy novels to my favorite comic books. Thank you, Mom, for taking me to Collage to buy my weekly comic books. My love for books opened my mind up to a world of possibility and eventually led to my creating something special of my own. Dad, thank you for the hundreds of books you've put in my lap at birthdays and Christmas. I'm already passing the love of reading on to my kids.

To my brothers from the same mother, Adrian and Michael Del Monte. We have an unbreakable bond, and I thank you both for always bringing me back to reality, keeping me humble, and inspiring me to be a real man. A special mention goes out to all the rest of my family for your interest in my weird world of muscle and marketing. I'm grateful I have each of you.

To my muscle-building mentors and coaches, Dr. John Berardi, Ian King, Matthew Craig, Murray Middlemost, Charles Poliquin, Ben Pakulski, the late Peter Chiasson, Eric Seifert, Ryan Faehnle, Wade Lightheart, Brandon Green, Joseph Bennett, Dr. Jacob Wilson, and Ryan Lowery. You each wow me with your expertise, passion, and brilliance.

To my past and present business mentors and coaches, Sandro Salsi, Craig Ballantyne, Bedros Keuillian, Eben Pagan, Mark Widamer, Dean Jackson, and Ryan Levesque. Each one of you helped lay the marketing foundation to make my ideas profitable. You have each had more impact on me than you know.

To Team Del Monte for taking this nonstop roller coaster ride with me through the years and bearing with my hundreds of always "urgent," last minute, "guaranteed breakthrough" ideas.

To Robin Colucci, my book coach, who got this book off the starting line and over the finish line. Your help and partnership on this book has been monumental. You underpromised and overdelivered and this book is equally yours as it is mine, I just get all the credit! Mille grazie.

To Yuri Elkaim, who introduced me to his incredible book agent Celeste Fine at Sterling Lord Literistic, who walked me through the book negotiating process and landed me a great deal. You both rock!

ACKNOWLEDGMENTS

To all the staff at Chapters bookstore in Ancaster, Ontario, for telling me every time I walked in there, "I'm waiting for your book, Mr. Vince!"

To Joel Marion, who helped me write the original book proposal for this book way back in 2009. Your level of generosity is above the rest, Brosef! Thank you James Villepigue for your generous insights, believing in my vision, and helping me move this project forward.

To the entire BenBella team. I'm truly honored to get to work alongside and learn from each one of your exceptional "super powers."

To the original "marketing" gangsters who all met up in West Palm Beach so many years ago with plans to rule the world. You each supported me at the very beginning and guaranteed my success, Jeff Anderson, Mike Geary, Jon Benson, Craig Ballantyne, Joey Atlas, Ryan Lee, Chris Guerriero, Chad Tackett, Scott Colby, and Jim Labadie.

To my incredible circle of Christian brothers living larger than ever—Joel Marion, Mike Westerdal, Shaun Hadsall, Ryan Colby, Dan Long, Mike Whitfield, Geoff Neupert, John Rowly, Jim Rowly, Chad Howse, Bruce Krahn, Todd Kuslikis, Dan Ritchie, Chris Wilson, Anthony Alayon, Charles Livingston, Vinnie Leone, Nate Hopkins, Joe Barton, Jeff Radich, Cody Sipe, and the leader of our group, the one and only Italian Stallion, my pops, Luciano Del Monte. I'm grateful for your love, encouragement, realness, resourcefulness, and never missing a single event in my life.

To Kory and Richard, for helping to market, promote, and make the entire world aware of this book and the message behind it and for putting up with my constant flow of "game changing" ideas.

To each and every influencer and leader who reviewed my book and wrote an endorsement.

To Arthur and Jo at Arsenik Studios for (both) the awesome photo shoots.

To Stephanie Matos, the ultimate fact-finder. Thanks for double-checking every single claim in this book.

To each one of my affiliates, you know who you are. If you've ever endorsed any of my programs over the years, I can't tell you how grateful I am by your support and sends.

To Team VIP (Vinny's Important People): If you read my newsletter, watch my YouTube videos, engage with my Facebook posts, and/or share my work, thank you. I'd like to offer my deepest gratitude for following my work, investing in my programs, betting on yourself, taking action, and getting outside of your comfort zone. I'm super pumped to see your 30-week "shock and awe" transformation pictures from my brand-new program. Gains without the gear, baby!

To my B.M.W. (beautiful, marvelous wife) Flavia, thank you for "living large" in your own life well before you met me and living larger than ever today. Thank you for being my #1 fan, best friend, and confidante. I'm so happy that we're doing life together and raising the two sweetest (sometimes) kids in the world! Ready to start working on #3?

Most importantly, none of this would be possible without God, my father in heaven. Thank you for blessing me beyond measure and enlarging my world.

CAN YOU HOOK A BROTHER UP?

THANK YOU FOR BUYING MY BOOK. Pat yourself on the back for taking action and betting on yourself. I'm super pumped to see your before and after pictures when you complete the program. There's no doubt you have 30 weeks of muscle-building greatness in your hands and are about to radically transform your body. Please send me your before and picture pictures along with your story to personal@vincedelmontefitness.com with the SUBJECT LINE "My 30-Week Living Large Transformation." I would love to share your story on my sites.

Now, I have a small favor to ask. Could you take just a few minutes and leave a comment on Amazon? I love hearing from the ambitious guys like you who follow my work, and it would be awesome to hear your feedback. I'm on a mission to help one million men build muscle by the year 2020, and this is a way that tracks my progress. Your feedback will inspire more men to take action and defeat their skinny genetics.

Also, be sure to tell your best buddy who also deserves to build a rock-solid body about this book. That would mean the world to me. Thanks again, I look forward to reading your comments, and hearing about your success.

To living larger than ever,

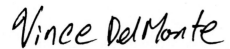

f facebook.com/vincedelmontelivelargetv

▶ youtube.com/vincedelmonte

📷 instagram.com/vincedelmonte

👻 vincedelmonte

TAKE THE NEXT STEP

CLAIM YOUR <u>FREE</u> 7-DAY TRIAL TO THE LIVE LARGE INNER CIRCLE TODAY!

I want to coach YOU with one mission, one goal, one focus: your leanest, strongest, and most muscular body ever . . . the no-nonsense way!

Led by Vince Del Monte and his personal inner circle of coaches and mentors, the Live Large Inner Circle is our private members' community where fellow members are always there to answer your questions and to help accelerate your transformation, so you don't have to go it alone. Inside, you will have the opportunity to receive personalized help and attend monthly "Anything Goes" coaching calls to ensure your fastest, safest, and easiest possible results, plus so much more. Be sure to claim your free 7-day trial inside the Live Large Inner Circle right now.

JOIN US AND START LIVING LARGER TODAY
GetLivingLarge.com/InnerCircle

ABOUT THE AUTHOR

Vince Del Monte's mission is to help one million men learn the most direct and efficient way to build muscle without the nonsense, and so far he has transformed tens of thousands of lives with his bestselling *No-Nonsense Muscle Building: Skinny Guy Secrets to Insane Muscle Gain*, which has sold more than 80,000 copies in over 120 countries. He's since gone on to create an entire suite of programs and live events to build a multi-million-dollar information business based around helping skinny guys build muscle the natural way. Vince received an Honors Kinesiology degree from the University of Western Ontario. He enjoys the natural bodybuilding and fitness lifestyle, and he has competed in over a dozen fitness model competitions and earned his Pro Card with the World Beauty Fitness and Fashion (WBFF) in 2011. Vince has been featured in *Men's Health, Men's Fitness, Maximum Fitness, Reps, Inside Fitness, World Physique, Iron Man, FitnessX,* and dozens of other online and offline publications. He lives in Ontario with his wife and two children.

ENDNOTES

1. By the time he was 11, Cutler was hefting 80-pound concrete forms while working for his brothers' concrete foundation business in Sterling, MA. "I was always the strongest kid," Cutler recalls. "The first time I went in the gym I benched 315 pounds—and I'd never lifted weights before." "Mister Muscle/Jay Cutler Profile." *For Him Magazine* (FHM), (2004). Retrieved from: http://andrewvontz.com/wp-content/uploads/2012/09/CLIPS-FHM-7-04-Jay-Cutler-Feature-Compressed-6.pdf

2. In 2013, health and fitness products represented 14 of the top 50 most frequently run long-form product infomercials, with Total Gym (a $799 home exercise bench) ranking #3. Lipozene (a weight loss product) ranked #1 in spending for short-form infomercials during the same period. http://money.usnews.com/money/personal-finance/articles/2013/01/02/the-heavy-price-of-losing-weight

3. G. B. Forbes et al, "Deliberate overeeding in women and men: energy cost and composition of the weight gain," *British Journal of Nutrition* 56, no. 1 (1986): 1-9.

4. Shape Up America! "Everything You Want to Know About Body Fat," www.shapeup.org/bfl/basics1.html.

5. R. H. Strauss, R. R. Lanese, and W. B. Malarkey, "Weight loss in amateur wrestlers and its effect on serum testosterone levels," JAMA 254, no. 23 (1985): 3337-38.

6. J. N. Roemmich and W. E. Sinning, "Weight loss and wrestling training: effects on growth-related hormones," *Journal of Applied Physiology* 82, no. 6 (1997): 1760-64.

7. E. B. Geer and W. Shen, "Gender differences in insulin resistance, body composition, and energy balance," *Gender Medicine* 6 (2009): 60-75.

8. B. B. Kahn and J. S. Flier, "Obesity and insulin resistance," *Journal of Clinical Investigation* 106, no. 4 (2000): 473.

9. Verne Harnish, *Mastering the Rockefeller Habits: What You Must Do to Increase the Value of Your Growing Firm* (Ashburn, VA: Gazelles, Inc., 2002).

10. David P. Swain and Clinton A. Brawner, *ACSM's Resource Manual for Guidelines for Exercise Testing and Prescription* (Philadelphia, PA: Lippincott Williams and Wilkins, 2012).

11. B. J. Schoenfeld, "The mechanisms of muscle hypertrophy and their application to resistance training," *The Journal of Strength and Conditioning Research* 24, no. 10 (2010): 2857-72.

12. M. Toigo and U. Boutellier, "New fundamental resistance exercise determinants of molecular and cellular muscle adaptations," *European Journal of Applied Physiology* 97 (2006): 643-63.

13. J. Vierck et al., "Satellite cell regulation following myotrauma caused by resistance exercise," *Cell Biology International* 24 (2000): 263-72.

14. S. E. Mulligan et al., "Influence of resistance exercise volume on serum growth hormone and cortisol concentrations in women," *Journal of Strength & Conditioning Research* 10 (1996): 256-62.

15. T. N. Shepstone et al., "Short-term high- vs. low-velocity isokinetic lengthening training results in greater hypertrophy of the elbow flexors in young men," *Journal of Applied Physiology* 98 (2005): 1768-76.

16. Y. Takarada, H. Takazawa, and N. Ishii, "Applications of vascular occlusion diminish disuse atrophy of knee extensor muscles," *Medicine & Science in Sports & Exercise* 32

17. http://baye.com/the-sun-tan-analogy
    http://www.leanandmuscular.org/3-things-you-must-know-to-build-muscle.php

18. Boullosa, D., & Nakamura, F. (2013). The evolutionary significance of fatigue. *Frontiers in Physiology*, 4, 309.

19. C. Garg, "Effects of isotonic (dynamic constant external resistance) eccentric strength training at various speeds on concentric and isometric strength of quadriceps muscle," *Indian Journal of Physiotherapy & Occupational Therapy* 3, no. 3 (2009): 24–30.

20. J. Vierck et al., "Satellite cell regulation following myotrauma caused by resistance exercise," *Cell Biology International*, 24 (2000): 263–72.

21. www.bettermovement.org/2010/seven-things-you-should-know-about-pain-science

22. Bi F. Bieuzen, C. M. Bleakley, and J. T. Costello, "Contrast water therapy and exercise-induced muscle damage: a systematic review and meta-analysis," *PloS One* 8, no. 4 (2013): e62356.

23. D. J. Cochrane, "Alternating hot and cold water immersion for athlete recovery: a review," *Physical Therapy in Sport* 5, no. 1 (2004): 26–32.

24. G. Howatson and K. A. Van Someren, "The prevention and treatment of exercise-induced muscle damage," *Sports Medicine* 38, no. 6 (2008): 483–503.

25. S. Y. Huang et al., "Short-duration massage at the hamstrings musculotendinous junction induces greater range of motion," *The Journal of Strength and Conditioning Research* 24, no. 7 (2010): 1917–24.

26. G. C. Goats, "Massage—the scientific basis of an ancient art; Part 1: The techniques," *British Journal of Sports Medicine* 28, no. 3 (1994): 149–52.

27. M. Hernandez-Rief, T. Field, and H. Theakston (2001). "Lower back pain is reduced and range of motion increased after massage therapy." *International Journal of Neuroscience*, 106(3-4), 131-145.

28. T. Field et al., "Lower back pain and sleep disturbance are reduced following massage therapy," *Journal of Bodywork and Movement Therapies* 11, no. 12 (2007): 141–45.

29. P. Weerapong and G. S. Kolt, "The mechanisms of massage and effects on performance, muscle recovery and injury prevention," *Sports Medicine* 35, no. 3 (2005): 235–56.

30. http://muscleactivation.com

31. www.forbes.com/sites/danmunro/2014/06/16/u-s-healthcare-ranked-dead-last-compared-to-10-other-countries

32. http://www.commonwealthfund.org/publications/press-releases/2014/jun/us-health-system-ranks-last

33. T.K. LaPier (1997), "Glucocorticoid-induced muscle atrophy. The role of exercise in treatment and prevention." *Journal of Cardiopulmonary Rehabilitation*, 17, 76–84

34. M. Ekstedt, T. Åkerstedt, and M. Söderström, "Microarousals during sleep are associated with increased levels of lipids, cortisol, and blood pressure," *Psychosomatic Medicine* 66, no. 6 (2004): 925–31.

35. K. Spiegel, R. Leproult, and E. Van Cauter, "Impact of sleep debt on metabolic and endocrine function," *The Lancet* 354, no. 9188 (1999): 1435–39.

36. M. P. St-Onge et al., "Sleep restriction increases the neuronal response to unhealthy food in normal-weight individuals," *International Journal of Obesity* 38, no. 3 (2014): 411-16.

37. P. A. Bryant, J. Trinder, and N. Curtis, "Sick and tired: does sleep have a vital role in the immune system?," *Nature Reviews Immunology* 4, no. 6 (2004): 457-67.

38. Harvard Health Publications, (2010-2016). Water, Sodium & Potassium: Guidelines to water, sodium & potassium intake. Retrieved from: http://www.health.harvard.edu/press_releases

39. M. Rondanelli et al., "The effect of melatonin, magnesium, and zinc on primary insomnia in long-term care facility residents in Italy: a double-blind, placebo-controlled clinical trial," *Journal of the American Geriatrics Society* 59, no. 1 (2011): 82-90.

40. "Magnesium," http://umm.edu/health/medical/altmed/supplement/magnesium

41. National Sleep Foundation, "Six tips to design the ideal bedroom for sleep," http://sleepfoundation.org/sleep-news/six-tips-design-the-ideal-bedroom-sleep

42. www.youtube.com/watch?v=igdwYFGBDW4

43. R. Van Gelder, "How the clock sees the light," *Nature Neuroscience* 11 (2008): 628-30.

44. National Sleep Foundation, "How much sleep do we really need?" http://sleepfoundation.org/how-sleep-works/how-much-sleep-do-we-really-need/page/0/1

45. S. Nissen et al., "Effect of leucine metabolite β-hydroxy-β-methylbutyrate on muscle metabolism during resistance-exercise training," *Journal of Applied Physiology* 81, no. 5 (1996): 2095-104.

46. J. F. Dorgan et al., "Effects of dietary fat and fiber on plasma and urine androgens and estrogens in men: a controlled feeding study," *The American Journal of Clinical Nutrition* 64, no. 6 (1996): 850-55.

47. www.nih.gov/researchmatters/september2013/09232013testosterone.htm

48. Iowa State University, "Carbohydrates," www.extension.iastate.edu/humansciences/content/carbohydrate

49. A. Papathanasopoulos and M. Camilleri, "Dietary fiber supplements: effects in obesity and metabolic syndrome and relationship to gastrointestinal functions," *Gastroenterology* 138, no. 1 (2010): 65-72.

50. C. Hull, R. S. Greco, and D. L. Brooks, "Alleviation of constipation in the elderly by dietary fiber supplementation," *Journal of the American Geriatrics Society* 28, no. 9 (1980): 410-14.

51. E. Giovannucci et al., "Intake of fat, meat, and fiber in relation to risk of colon cancer in men," *Cancer Research* 54, no. 9 (1994): 2390-97.

52. U.S. Geological Survey, "The water in you," http://water.usgs.gov/edu/propertyyou.html

53. H. H. Mitchell et al., "The chemical composition of the adult human body and its bearing on the biochemistry of growth," *Journal of Biological Chemistry* 158 (1945): 625-37.

54. A. Jeukendrup and M. Gleeson, *Sport Nutrition, 2nd ed.* (Champaign, IL: Human Kinetics, 2010).

55. B. Halliwell, K. Zhao, and M. Whiteman, "The gastrointestinal tract: a major site of antioxidant action?," *Free Radical Research* 33, no. 6 (2000): 819-30.

56. R. D. Hurt et al., "Nutritional status of a group of alcoholics before and after admission to an alcoholism treatment unit," *The American Journal of Clinical Nutrition* 34, no. 3 (1981): 386-92.

57. M.A. Emanuele and N. Emanuele, *Alcohol and the Male Reproductive System*, http://pubs.niaaa.nih.gov/publications/arh25-4/282-287.htm

58. S. Q. Siler, R. A. Neese, and M. K. Hellerstein, "De novo lipogenesis, lipid kinetics, and whole-body lipid balances in humans after acute alcohol consumption," *The American Journal of Clinical Nutrition* 70, no. 5 (1999): 928–36.

59. M. S. Cook, *The Phytozyme Cure: Treat or Reverse More Than 30 Serious Health Conditions with Powerful Plant Nutrients* (Malden, MA: John Wiley and Sons, 2010).

60. Encyclopedia Britannica, (2015). Human aging: Physiology and sociology. Retrieved from: http://www.britannica.com/science/human-aging

61. E. Howell, *Enzyme Nutrition: The Food Enzyme Concept* (Penguin, 1995).

62. G. A. Kleter, A. A. Peijnenburg, and H. J. Aarts, "Health considerations regarding horizontal transfer of microbial transgenes present in genetically modified crops," *BioMed Research International* 4 (2005): 326–52.

63. S. M. Snedeker and A. G. Hay, "Do interactions between gut ecology and environmental chemicals contribute to obesity and diabetes?," *Environmental Health Perspectives* 120, no. 3 (2011): 332–39.

64. M. S. Palmnäs et al., "Low-dose aspartame consumption differentially affects gut microbiota-host metabolic interactions in the diet-induced obese rat," *PLoS One* 9, no. 10 (2014): e109841.

65. www.cornucopia.org/Yogurt-docs/CultureWars-FullReport.pdf

66. T. A. Churchward-Venne, N. A. Burd, and S. M. Phillips, "Nutritional regulation of muscle protein synthesis with resistance exercise: strategies to enhance anabolism," *Nutrition & Metabolism* 9, no. 1 (2012): 40.

67. J. E. Chavarro et al., "Soy food and isoflavone intake in relation to semen quality parameters among men from an infertility clinic," *Human Reproduction* 23, no. 11 (2008): 2584–90.

68. K. S. Weber et al., "Dietary soy-phytoestrogens decrease testosterone levels and prostate weight without altering LH, prostate 5 alpha-reductase or testicular steroidogenic acute regulatory peptide levels in adult male Sprague-Dawley rats," *Journal of Endocrinology* 170 (2001): 591–99.

69. J. M. Joy et al., "The effects of 8 weeks of whey or rice protein supplementation on body composition and exercise performance," *Nutrition Journal* 12, no. 1 (2013): 86.

70. X. S. Wang et al., "Characterization, amino acid composition and in vitro digestibility of hemp (Cannabis sativa L.) proteins," *Food Chemistry* 107, no. 1 (2008): 11–18.

71. C. H. Tang et al., "Physicochemical and functional properties of hemp (Cannabis sativa L.) protein isolate," *Journal of Agricultural and Food Chemistry* 54, no. 23 (2006): 8945–50.

72. X. S. Wang et al., "Characterization, amino acid composition and in vitro digestibility of hemp (Cannabis sativa L.) proteins," *Food Chemistry* 107, no. 1 (2008): 11–18.

73. C. T. Lin and B. S. Haiming, "The research of hempseed protein powder on nutritional physiological functions of growing rats," *Journal of Chinese Institute of Food Science and Technology* 2 (2011): 017.

74. G. Keller and J. Papasan, *The ONE Thing* (Austin, TX: Bard Press, 2013), 191.